The
L+ng Life
Equati−n

First published in North America by Adams Media, an F+W Publications Company
57 Littlefield Street
Avon, MA 02322
www.adamsmedia.com

Conceived and produced by
Elwin Street Productions
144 Liverpool Road
London N1 1LA
www.elwinstreet.com

ISBN 10: 1-59869-813-3
ISBN 13: 978-1-59869-813-8

Layouts designed by Louise Leffler

Picture credits:
Bigstock: 11, 61; Corbis: 81, 94; Dreamstime: 12, 17, 26, 31, 33, 79, 101, 127; Getty Images: 21, 25, 73, 87, 105, 125; istockphoto: 19, 28, 32, 35, 37, 40. 43, 46, 48, 50, 53, 55, 63, 65, 74, 77, 83, 85, 90, 92, 99, 102, 106, 109, 112, 123, 128, 131, 134, 135.

Printed in Singapore
J I H G F E D C B A

This book is available at quantity discounts for bulk purchases.
For information, please call 1-800-289-0963.

The
L+ng Life
Equati-n

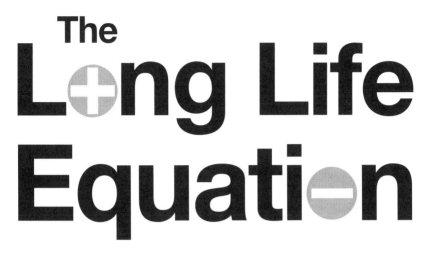

Trisha MacNair M.D., M.A.
with Olga Calof M.D.

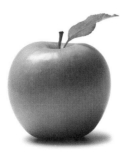

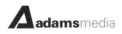

Contents

Introduction

Can you add years to your life? Good genes, habits, and attitude all combine to play a role in longevity. If you adopt a positive, active lifestyle, chances are you can add many healthy, happy years to your life. So what are the ingredients in this recipe for success? *The Long Life Equation* offers 100 factors that can add or subtract years from your life. Fifty-six of these are the "best practices" to emulate. The other 44 can subtract years from your life. The rest is up to you.

The U.S. Census Bureau estimates that by the year 2050, there may be over 800,000 centenarians in our midst. Would you like to be one of them? While genetics does play a part in longevity, a healthy lifestyle along with a positive outlook can help to extend your life.

As an endocrinologist, one health habit most prominent in my advice to every patient I see is prevention. In my practice, I see many diabetic patients with severe, debilitating complications of the disease who may have had a chance of preventing the complications. Prevention doesn't just mean getting regular checkups (although they are definitely part of the equation), but also staying physically active, emotionally healthy, aware of your environment, avoiding disease through information, prevention and vaccination and making the right lifestyle choices.

Modern medicine has some miracles to offer. Doctors have tools to help prevent colon cancer, cervical cancer, heart attacks, and strokes. We can be coaches to life improvement; we can be your partners in health. With early diagnosis and treatment of some illnesses, like diabetes, we can prevent complications.

There is one important common theme to this book: how to live a long, happy, satisfying life. You can do it by thinking sensibly about how to maintain, or improve your health, outlook, and lifestyle. Will following this book make you live to 100? I hope so. But what this book cannot control is your genetic predisposition or other, unknown risks such as accidents.

The best result of reading this book is this: that you find yourself looking at the world in a new way, a world in which you are happier, healthier and living longer!

Olga Calof, M.D.

How to use this book

This book is filled with information based on recent international medical evidence and published research which spells out the risks and benefits of many factors known to influence health and longevity. But even when a factor has been clearly shown to cut or prolong lifespan, it can be difficult to know the exact implications for an individual.

To give you some idea of the importance of each factor to your chances of living a long and healthy life, we have used medical knowledge and experience with patients to scrutinize the results of the research and provide a rough guide that sums up its effects in terms of the years that it might add or remove to an individual's lifespan. When the science behind the years is particularly controversial we have added a "?" motif.

Start with an average life span of 70 years, and add or subtract the years for each factor outlined as they pertain to you, and you might get a picture of how long you could expect to live. But please don't take the result too seriously—it is no more than an estimate. Life and health is far too complex for any rational scientist to be able to predict exactly how much of it could be attributed to any single factor in one person. The Years guide should be seen as food for thought, to help you understand the influences on mortality, rather than a reliable guarantee of what will definitely happen. No matter how much information we have, none of us can know for sure the exact moment of our death but we can build a picture in our minds of the kind of risks to a long and healthy life that we face, and use this to improve our wellbeing.

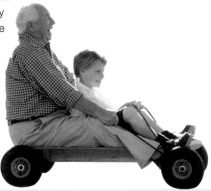

Could you live forever?

20 questions to predict your chances of living a long life

Part One: Mental Well-being
Which answers most closely match your thoughts?

1. When I think about my future:
a. I feel optimistic and want to make exciting plans.
b. I feel too old to look forward to things.
c. I don't even think about the years to come.

2. In the community I live in:
a. there are lots of people I know through the sports or other activities I am involved in, and I feel I belong.
b. I don't really get involved and I sometimes feel very lonely.
c. I do get involved now and then, and have a few friends.

3. About my spiritual beliefs:
a. I have a strong religious faith that is important to me.
b. I don't really know what I believe in.
c. I have spiritual beliefs but I don't attend services regularly.

4. My daily stress levels are:
a. Stress? What stress?
b. overwhelming. I'm constantly feeling on edge.
c. manageable—I have some stress but keep on top of it.

Part Two: Physical Well-being
Which answer most closely describes you?

5. In my family:
a. there is no recognizable pattern of inherited disease.
b. there is a strong history of either cancer; heart or blood vessel disease; degenerative diseases of the nerves and brain; or diabetes.
c. a few people have died at a relatively young age of similar problems listed in option b.

6. In my diet:
a. there are freshly prepared, healthy meals full of fresh fruit and vegetables.
b. there are plenty of chips and candy.
c. there is healthy food when I can get it, but quite often I rely on pre-packaged instant meals.

7. I regularly take:
a. Omega-3 supplements.
b. my car to the pub.
c. a look at articles in the papers on healthy eating.

8. Exercise is:
a. a vital part of my daily routine.
b. something I avoid as much as possible.
c. something I ought to do more.

Part Three: Environment
Which answer most closely describes you or your views?

9. I live:
a. in the countryside.
b. in the middle of a city.
c. in the suburbs of a medium-sized town.

10. Pollution from chemicals, radiation, and other potentially harmful substances:
a. is a constant threat to my health that I take active steps to guard against.
b. is something that scaremongers and the media go on about—I don't really believe in it.
c. is something I mean to check up about but haven't got around to yet.

11. I wash my hands:
a. several times a day, especially before eating.
b. never—I can't see the point.
c. now and then.

12. My home:
a. has been thoroughly checked for safety hazards and fire risks.
b. is a death trap.
c. could be tidier and safer.

Part Four: Dealing with Disease

Which answer most closely describes you, your habits, and your health?

13. Screening tests such as blood pressure tests, dental check-ups, and pap smear tests:
a. are important and something I always attend.
b. are mostly not really worth bothering with.
c. are something I occasionally go for.

14. Heart disease is:
a. something that I personally take particular steps to avoid.
b. not something that will happen to me.
c. something I worry about but don't do much about yet.

15. My blood pressure is:
a. normal or lower than normal.
b. probably high—I never measure it.
c. rising fast as I answer these questions.

16. Exercise, antioxidants, fiber, and masses of fruit and vegetables are a recipe for:
a. avoiding cancer—I follow this recipe.
b. someone else but not me—sounds far too dreary.
c. avoiding cancer—if only I followed it!

Part Five: Choices and Risks

Which answer most closely describes you and your lifestyle?

17. I:
a. have never smoked.
b. currently smoke every day.
c. used to smoke but gave up at least six months ago.

18. I drink:
a. 0 to 2 units of alcohol a day.
b. no alcohol some days but a lot (more than 10 units) on other days.
c. an average of 3 to 4 units of alcohol a day but rarely more than this.

19. Car racing, downhill skiing, hang-gliding, or scuba diving are:
a. just too frightening for me.
b. lots of fun—I do these sorts of sports whenever I can.
c. something I'll do now and then.

20. My job:
a. is office based—it's very quiet.
b. is very dangerous—there are lots of risks involved.
c. can have difficult moments but doesn't usually expose me to dangers.

Scoring

Score 2 for every "a" answer
Score 0 for every "b" answer
Score 1 for every "c" answer

Results

0–13: Whoa! Look out! You could meet an early death unless you start putting some of the advice in this book to work.

14–24: You are doing well but still have more to do if you really want to live a longer, healthier life.

27+: Well done! You stand a good chance of living a long life, because you seem to know a lot about keeping healthy.

Can feeling good help you live longer? Or do years of negative emotions, stress, and sadness cut it short? The links are complex and not well understood. Where physical health is measurable—we can monitor blood pressure levels to ensure they remain within a healthy range, or link daily cigarette habits to mortality statistics—the good and harmful effects of emotions are far harder to gauge. One person's idea of happiness might be very different to another's.

In some ways, it's clear that mental well-being promotes longevity. The more of that "feel-good" factor you have, the better you are likely to do at work, for example, and the more money you are likely to earn, so you can buy healthier food, afford to go to the gym, and take relaxing holidays. You are also more likely to work better in a team, and get on well with others. Happy people make more friends, have better relationships, and are more likely to find long-lasting love and a stable marriage. All these things contribute to a longer life. Mental well-being is not only valuable because it feels good, but also because it has beneficial consequences. And happiness begets happiness: the better you feel, the better you do—and this in turn makes you feel even better!

PART ONE

Mental Well-being

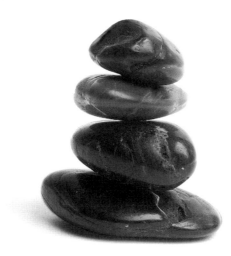

Thinking old

— 5 YEARS

Thinking old is the quickest step to speeding up your demise. Take a tip from those people who don't even let the idea into their head. You don't have to squeeze yourself into the latest dance gear or save up for cosmetic surgery—just keep an open mind to life's endless possibilities.

Relish new challenges, learn new skills, and set new goals. Embrace new technology, and use what you need from it. Scorn convention—if there is something that you really want to do then find a way to do it. Never utter the words "I'm too old" (sometimes this might be true, but just don't dwell on it!). Why talk about your age? Once you're over 18 no one needs to know it. And never use phrases like "In my day…"—today is your day as much as anyone else's!

In keeping with the trend for women living longer than men (see entry 24), the oldest person ever is a woman. Jeanne-Louise Calment holds the Guinness World Record, having lived 122 years and 164 days. She was born in France in 1875 and she died in 1997. She was already 14 when the Eiffel Tower was completed in 1889 and was still riding a bicycle at 100. At the age of 114 she portrayed herself in the film Vincent and Me, in order to become the oldest actress in film.

2

Happiness
9 YEARS +

Low levels of life satisfaction have been linked with mortality, while other research has found that happy people act in healthier ways, getting more exercise and taking part in more social activities than unhappy people do. Positive emotions mean quicker recovery from illness and injury, a longer life, and less chance of disability.

Happiness may boost the immune system by increasing the number of immune cells available to fight viruses and bacteria. In one study conducted by Cohen, Doyle, Turner, Alper, and Skoner in 2003, the least happy third of the participants were 2.9 times more likely to develop a cold than the happiest. And cancer patients who experience more positive emotions each day have higher levels of "natural killer" cells (which can destroy cancer cells) or lower levels of stress hormones such as epinephrine and cortisol, which are known to be toxic to the immune system.

How to get happy

- Make a list of the sources of unhappiness in your life and look for ways to deal with these.

- Make a list of the real joys in your life and aim for a daily dose of one or more of them.

- Adopt the art of mindfulness. This form of meditation teaches you how to take pleasure from the simple things in life, even in daily chores—the warmth of soapy water as you wash up, or the color of a daisy as you walk to work.

- Set yourself realistic goals and expectations—you are less likely to be happy if you are chasing an impossible dream.

Optimism

✚ 8 YEARS

A well-known study by the Mayo Clinic in the early 1950s showed that optimists live about 8 years longer on average than pessimists. More recently they have also shown that optimists are 50 percent less likely to die prematurely.

Optimistic older people have better immune function than pessimistic old people, so being hopeful may keep disease at bay. Optimism also helps you to deal with illness, while pessimists tend to believe that "nothing I do will matter" and are more passive about their health. Research has shown that optimism is very helpful in heart disease, for example, lowering the likelihood of angina and heart attacks. Similarly, hope is a powerful weapon for cancer patients, and can significantly increase how long someone survives.

How to become an optimist

What to avoid	What to do
• Learn to recognize and abandon negative forms of thinking. • Avoid filtering (focusing only on negative things) and personalizing (blaming yourself for bad things). • Avoid catastrophizing (always expecting the worst) and polarizing (seeing things as always good or bad, not shades of either).	• Work hard at taking a more positive view on life. • Look for the good things, no matter how small, and cherish them. • Try to play down the bad things—deal with them and move on. • Keep company with optimists and hope their attitude rubs off on you!

Low self-esteem
4 YEARS —

Low self-esteem can gnaw away at life. People with higher levels of self-esteem value themselves more and so put more effort into looking after their health and well-being. They also tend to be happier (see entry 2) people. These are two reasons why self-esteem is linked to a longer life. A study of nursing-home residents who were equally physically healthy found that the higher their self-esteem and the less depressed they were, the longer they lived.

There are positive steps you can take to build up your self-esteem if it is at a low ebb. Start by making a list of your good points, and don't be hard on yourself. Once you have your list it is important to abandon modesty and congratulate yourself frequently on these points every day.

Another great way to boost your self-image is to learn a new skill—origami, playing the saxophone, skydiving—it really doesn't matter which you choose, but take it seriously and practice it until you can do it well in order to get the most benefit from it.

Doing something nice for others has been shown to increase our self-esteem—find a community group you can volunteer with, preferably one that interests you. The chance to polish your halo on a regular basis by helping others is one of the most powerful ways to build self-esteem.

Finally, hang out with the right people and ignore or avoid people who threaten your self-esteem by being negative or acting more superior than you. Once you are in with the right crowd, embrace their company as it will have huge benefits to how good you feel about yourself.

5

Conscientiousness
✚ **2 YEARS**

Conscientiousness has been shown to be associated with a longer, healthier life. The Terman Life-Cycle Study, which ran from 1922 to 1991, found that adults who weren't very conscientious during their childhood died at a younger age.

Conscientiousness is related to emotional intelligence and involves being thoughtful, thorough, organized, and committed. It can make a person more aware of their own health needs, and more likely to take a serious view of the prevention of disease. This characteristic also tends to be visible in harder-working and more reliable individuals. For instance, conscientious people are more likely to get vaccinated or have regular physical exams and screening tests, exercise even when they don't feel like it, eat healthy foods when they would really rather eat a bar of chocolate, and avoid risk-taking activities such as drinking, drugs, and dangerous sports, because they are concerned about the effects on themselves as well as on those around them. Furthermore, conscientiousness in students has been related to higher academic achievement.

Being conscientious may also develop into care for others and the community, which builds stability and support in your own life as well as in the lives of others. A conscientious person is also more likely to react constructively and positively to emotional and social challenges, and is more likely to create work and living environments that promote good health.

Having faith

7 YEARS +

In virtually every one of more than a thousand studies examining the effects of spirituality on healing, a powerful link was found between faith and longevity. A 12-year study at the University of Iowa, for example, found that those who attended religious services at least once a week were 35 percent more likely to live longer than those who never attended a church or other faith-based events.

Being actively involved in a spiritual community—by going to church or the mosque regularly, for example—boosts the immune system and helps to keep high blood pressure and clogged arteries at bay. It is associated with lower levels of Interleukin-6, a mediator of inflammation linked to age-related diseases such as atherosclerosis. Researchers speculate that this positive effect is the result of a more healthy diet and lifestyle among churchgoers. The strong sense of community that most religions offer may also play a part.

Religious leaders, on the other hand, pragmatically suggest that going to church won't protect you from all the horrible things that happen in life, but will give you the strength to tackle and overcome them.

Marriage

+ # 7 YEARS

Both men and women live healthier, wealthier, happier, and longer lives when they are in a stable partnership. There is a huge amount of research showing a strong link between supportive social relationships and well-being. In most societies, getting married is one of the main ways to establish this sort of intense and stable relationship.

In 2006, scientists from the University of California, Los Angeles, confirmed that married couples are more likely to live to an old age than their divorced, widowed, or unmarried counterparts. Their research showed that people who never marry are almost two-thirds more likely to die early, even though they appeared to be in better physical shape than their peers.

People who are happily married are less likely to have financial difficulties or physical or mental health problems than those who aren't married. When illness does strike, being married may help speed recovery: married people have been shown to have higher survival rates than single, widowed, or divorced people in some cancer cases, for example.

It appears there is something about marriage—a sense of belonging to a social institution, perhaps, or a public demonstration of shared aspirations— that gives it the edge over cohabitation. As for gay partnerships, although it is likely that a settled partnership might bring the same sort of health benefits that married heterosexuals enjoy, it is too early to guess at the effect of marriage in this context as gay marriages have only recently been permitted in some countries.

Divorce

3 YEARS —

Divorce can exact a greater, and in many cases longer-lasting, emotional and physical toll on former spouses than virtually any other life stress. Recent studies indicate that divorced adults have higher rates of emotional disturbance; accidental death; and death from heart disease, cancer, pneumonia, high blood pressure; and cirrhosis of the liver.

The divorced also have higher rates of admission to psychiatric hospitals and clinics, and make more visits to physicians than people who are married, single, or widowed. Men have a harder time living alone and if they have not remarried in six years, their rates of car accidents, alcoholism, drug abuse, depression, and anxiety increase.

But in very unhappy marriages, divorce eventually brings better health and a reduction in stress. Remarriage rates are high: 75 percent of divorced women and 80 percent of divorced men remarry, and those who form new romantic relationships may regain the lost years and happiness.

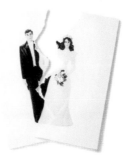

9

Young mothers

— 2 YEARS

On the one hand, the demands of having children may seem to cause gray hair and wrinkles as they suck every atom of your reserves. But they can also bring deep joy—that happiness factor that is so well linked to longevity.

What studies of large families in Utah have shown is that women who have more children live less long than those with smaller families, and that those who have their children late in life live longer. Men in this study seemed to be slightly less affected by the size or timing of their family.

Research among the Sami women of Finland, meanwhile, has found no link to family size, but showed that women who had their last child at an older age lived longest.

Evolutionary biologists call this the "Grandmother effect," whereby women have evolved to live until their children have successfully reproduced. Once they have helped their children through the difficulties of creating their own family (where, as the grandmother, they play an invaluable role in both teaching their child how to look after her new-born and in taking an active role in caring for their grandchild), their mortality rises steeply. So if you have your last child late and then encourage that child to do the same, you might gain yourself a few years!

Community
6 YEARS +

Human beings are inherently social creatures—our minds and bodies were designed to work best when we live together in a group and support each other through the normal stresses of life, whether simply gathering food or facing an enemy. Being isolated, on the other hand, especially after divorce or the death of a partner, is linked to an increased risk of depression and personal neglect, among other factors significantly linked to mortality.

Supportive social relationships improve your well-being: people who are more involved in their community have a better social support network, which helps them stay healthier and live longer than those who live alone.

How to get involved

- Join a club and meet people who share your interests.

- Go regularly to the local gym or sports center.

- Volunteer—start doing things for others and everyone will want to be your friend!

- Use local shops and services, and get to know your area well.

- Spend some time walking or just enjoying the buzz around you in a nearby park or nature reserve.

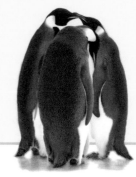

Stress

2 YEARS

Stress is the thread that pulls together a web of factors that affect your mortality—you could lose a year of your life for every major stressful event you tussle with, such as serious accidents or relationship crises.

The reason for this is that when you feel stressed your brain senses danger: Its "fight or flight" response urges into action various mechanisms in your body—releasing epinephrine, and raising your heart rate and blood pressure, for example, as well as unleashing the stress hormone called cortisol. This process is very helpful at the instant you need to confront a threat, but if stress persists in the long term, it can start to cause damage to the body. For instance, cortisol makes nerve cells take in calcium; if these cells become overloaded with calcium, they fire off signals too frequently and die—they are literally excited to death.

Some research has shown that raised cortisol levels seem to kill cells within the hippocampus, an area of the brain that controls memory. Cortisol also reduces the

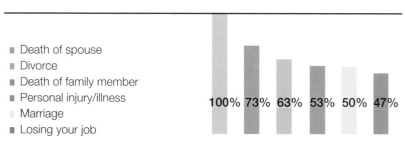

Event   **Stress level 100%**

- Death of spouse
- Divorce
- Death of family member
- Personal injury/illness
- Marriage
- Losing your job

100% 73% 63% 53% 50% 47%

brain's ability to make new neurons or nerve cells, and can generally cause premature aging of the brain. In addition, it changes the fats in the blood, which, combined with raised blood pressure, greatly increases the risk of a heart attack or stroke, and may also have a negative effect on the immune system.

So it is important to deal with the stress in your life as this will improve your health and longevity in a myriad of ways.

Easier said than done, the key to reducing stress is recognizing what causes it. Look at all the situations in your life, from work to relationships, family and health, and try to identify areas which regularly cause you anxiety. Simply identifying the stresses in your life is a positive step in itself. Equally, accepting that some degree of stress is a normal part of life is another step in the right direction.

In order to prevent stress you need to work out which stresses you think you could cut down. Start by looking at different areas of your life again: home, work, your relationships, or your finances, for example and think about what you can do to reduce the stressful situations that occur.

Some people use negative stress-management techniques such as denial, overeating, binge drinking, taking drugs, and smoking. Avoid these as much as possible as they are short-term solutions.

What you need to do is find positive stress-management techniques that suit you, such as taking time out for artistic expression, relaxation, massage techniques, exercise, or talking problems through with a friend or a therapist.

Good work-life balance

+ ## 3 YEARS?

While some people thrive on a demanding schedule and need a challenging occupation in their life, others find that a high-octane career leads only to burn-out, stress and depression. Everyone is different and it is important to recognize this. Ultimately, the key is balance—and only you know where the balance lies.

Find the right job for you—have a career assessment if you think that will help. Whether you prefer to spend your time pruning plants in a nursery or piloting a jumbo jet, you need to make sure your choice of work blends in with the other important areas of your life.

How to strike a good work-life balance

- Make a regular, honest appraisal of your job. Ask yourself if you look forward to work, or if your job limits the other things you want to do in life.

- Discuss problems at work before they overwhelm you. Speak to your manager about career progression and make the most of career advice provided by your company.

- If your work is starting to get you down, remember: it's never too late to stop and retrain in a new career.

- Don't forget that good communication is absolutely vital. Always be open with your family or partner about the ups and downs of your career to help balance your needs with theirs as well as to talk through your anxieties.

Social status

4 YEARS +

Social class can be a prickly issue, but overwhelming evidence points to longer lives for people with a higher social standing, rank, or position. It's called Status Syndrome and, according to epidemiologist Sir Michael Marmot, the pattern is repeated across all groups in society, all around the world, from the most disenfranchised to the leaders of our nations.

It's difficult to explain why status keeps us going. The links between social class—which contributes to status—and life expectancy are strong and becoming stronger. By the end of the twentieth century, professionals such as doctors and lawyers could expect to live, on average, nearly 1,500 days longer than unskilled manual workers. Key factors may include a feeling of having control over one's life, the ability to participate fully in society, and the connection between being rich and feeling rich. Whatever the mechanism, scientists have found that people with low social status are biologically older than their fancier peers, as their genetic material or DNA is shortened or becomes more frayed.

Exercise

+ # 2 YEARS

The effects of regular exercise on mental well-being alone could add as much as two or more years to your life. The Harvard Alumni Study, which took into account more than 71,000 men who had graduated from Harvard University and the University of Pennsylvania between 1916 and 1954, found that those men who regularly burned 2,000 calories a week while exercising lived, on average, two years longer than those who who chose to live a sedentary life.

Exercise works its magic because it is good for almost every system in the body. Although most of its effects are on physical health (take a deeper look at this in Part Two), it also works wonders on the psyche. People who exercise several times a week, whether to a moderate or intense degree, have lower levels of stress, anger, anxiety, and depression, all of which are linked to problems such as heart disease and an early death.

The bonus is that once you experience greater mental well-being, you are even more likely to engage in physical activity. So drag yourself out of that couch-potato rut, and you'll find it gets easier and easier to exercise and add years to your life.

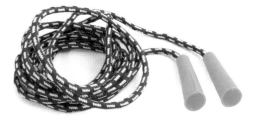

Clutter

1 YEAR? —

Creative clutter is one thing, but most people feel oppressed, stressed, and depressed when they are surrounded by chaos. The stress of clutter is a powerful subliminal force that surreptitiously drives your autonomic nervous system, whether the mess is a jumble of material possessions, a muddle of outstanding debts, or the turmoil of a tumultuous relationship.

Clutter can cause the pulse rate and blood pressure to simmer higher than is healthy, while epinephrine and cortisol do their damage. Figure out what kind of clutter you need to tackle, then get to work!

How to de-clutter

Clutter doesn't appear overnight and won't go away quickly either. Set aside time to sort out every aspect of your life. If it's a messy space you're faced with, for example:

- Break down the mess into small chunks: tackle a room, a cabinet, or even a drawer at a time.

- Reorganize your storage space so that you can put things away and then easily find them again.

- Get rid of stuff you haven't touched in years—bring it to a charity shop, give it to a friend, or have a garage sale.

- Get help: invite a friend over to help you sort the junk from the jewels!

- Choose a peaceful evening to sort out your finances, and if they look too chaotic to sort out yourself, get help from a financial advisor.

Laughter

+ # 1 YEAR?

You might instinctively imagine that laughing a lot has to be good for you and would surely help you to live longer.

Though research hasn't yet been able to conclusively prove this, laboratory experiments do suggest that being exposed to comedy may slightly improve your immunity to disease or reduce the amount of pain you feel. However, despite the fact that laughter is often used as a way to defuse stress, there is little evidence that it can actually improve physical health in the long run.

But don't be put off, you should certainly try to get a regular dose of giggles — jokes and tickling both have the desired effect — because having fun definitely makes you feel good and improves the overall quality of your life. There is even humor therapy and clown therapy, laughter yoga and laughter clubs for those who find it difficult to bring laughter into their lives spontaneously. Don't feel you have to become a comedian, though — the statistics show that, like other entertainers, comics have a tendency to die young (see entry 98).

Pets
2 YEARS +

All you need is love, and even the love of a tarantula or a goldfish might do. Having a pet that you can talk to and interact with may add years to your life. People with pets visit their doctors less and are less likely to suffer from depression.

Studies have found that stroking or being near a familiar animal can lower heart rates and blood pressure levels. One New York study looked at male and female stockbrokers already taking medication to control high blood pressure. Those with pets had significantly lower heart rate and blood pressure levels, which didn't become so raised when they were asked to do mental arithmetic and other stressful tests. This was particularly marked when the pet was nearby during the stressful event, when there was just half the increase in blood pressure compared with participants who did not own a pet.

Another New York study, conducted by Allen, Blascovich, and Mendes in 2002, reported that, after suffering a heart attack, those people who owned a dog were six times more likely to be alive one year later than those who didn't.

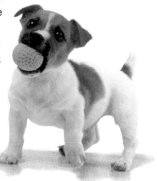

A pet may bring you new friends, too. People find companionship and comfort not just from the pets themselves, but also because they are more likely to engage with others because of owning the animal.

Depression

5 YEARS

Depression is like a gray blanket that smothers life. Different people mean different things by the word "depression," but a true clinical depression is linked to a lack of happiness and hopefulness, and an increase in anxiety or stress. Depression robs a person of motivation and gets in the way of decision-making. As a result, a depressed person is more likely to have low self-esteem, be unemployed, or have low career satisfaction, be isolated from society with poorer social relationships, and have less money to spend. This person is also more likely to engage in unhealthy habits such as smoking, drinking, and failing to take the medical treatments they need—each one a factor that influences longevity. In chronic severe depression, the deeper the mood the greater the chances the person will die young.

We don't fully understand how depression affects the body's natural defenses against disease, but it seems to interfere with the immune system in a variety of ways. For instance, depression can reduce the activity of cells in the body that are important in fighting off bacteria and viruses.

Studies have shown that depression can interfere with recovery from illness— holding back a patient from getting active again after surgery, for example—and reduce survival time among patients with serious conditions such as coronary heart disease.

The evidence that depression may play a part in cancer is slightly more controversial, but some studies have shown that it may help to increase the risk of cancer and speed up how fast the cancer progresses. Among people undergoing treatment for cancer, mood and level of depression are the strongest psychological predictors of how long an individual is likely to survive. Part of the explanation may simply be that a diagnosis of an aggressive, difficult-to-treat tumor with a poor prognosis is also more likely to make a person depressed, but depression does seem to have a separate effect, reducing a person's ability to cope with unpleasant treatments and fight their disease.

In older age, depression can spur on mental decline, leaving a person less able to look after themselves and increasing the risk of falls, accidents, malnourishment, infections, and other health problems. People with a history of clinical depression also have an increased risk of eventually developing specific types of dementia such as Alzheimer's disease, which are known to shorten life considerably.

There are many things you can do yourself to help beat depression, including exercise, which has been shown to reverse the effects of depression on the immune system, a healthy, well-balanced diet, plenty of good-quality rest, and a supportive network of friends, family, and local community.

Major depression is a serious medical condition—if you have a persistent low mood which disrupts sleep, interferes with your ability to get on with normal daily activities at home and at work, or leaves you feeling desperate about the future, get professional advice to sort it out. Your doctor will be able to talk to you about the different types of treatment available and what might be the most suitable course of action for you.

Meditation

✚ 3 YEARS

Take a tip from Eastern cultures, where meditation has been recommended for centuries as a natural path to health and longevity. The psychological benefits of meditation are now being more widely recognized the world over and are even used in some hospitals to reduce stress associated with chronic or terminal illness.

Studies of techniques such as transcendental meditation have shown that they can be effective in controlling blood pressure, keeping the arteries healthy, and reducing the risk of heart disease. It can also be used for personal development and to focus the mind.

How meditation helps you to live longer isn't clear but is probably related to a reduction in stress and its harmful effects. Those who meditate regularly say that it gives them an overall sense of peace and tranquillity, which may be as restorative as sleep, and helps them escape from the pressures of a busy life.

Meditation can lift mood, dispel anxiety, and be used to banish negative thoughts and pessimism. People who meditate regularly also say that it helps them focus and concentrate, improving their performance at work and bringing harmony to their relationships.

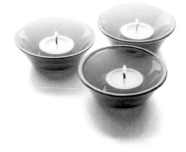

Active mind
4 YEARS ✚

Books can keep you alive! The more formal your education as a child, the better your memory and learning ability will persist into old age, keeping you more able to look after yourself and stay healthy.

But don't stop learning once you leave school. Keep stretching your mind, as learning forces the brain to grow new connections between the nerve cells—a direct antidote to aging. Pick up that electric guitar you have always wanted to play, learn ten pin bowling or how to become an expert at growing pumpkins. Even a simple change in routine—cooking a new recipe or taking a different route home from work, for instance—can help to keep your brain on its toes.

In an ongoing study started in 1993 by Rush University Medical Center in Chicago, for example, those who said that they spent time on activities involving significant information processing (such as listening to the radio, reading newspapers, going to museums, doing crosswords, or solving puzzle games) had nearly half the risk of developing Alzheimer's disease as those who did not.

And if you keep your mind active as you get older, you are more likely to keep your body active, too, and avoid the onset of dementia and other related conditions (see entry 92).

Sudoku

			2		9	4	3	1
8	1			6				
9	2		5	4		8		
	6		9		2		4	
			4	1		5		
			1					8
2					7			
	5			2		9	7	

The moment you are conceived, you are dealt a certain set of cards for life. Those cards—your genes—will have a myriad of powerful influences on how well and how long you live. They will, in part at least, determine how tall you grow, how smart you are, and how vulnerable to disease you will be.

But don't let this make you shut this book in a fit of hopeless despair, convinced that any effort to alter your genetic destiny is pointless. While you can't change your genetic make-up, you can learn how to play those cards as well as possible, by understanding what they mean for your physical well-being and how they could affect your future. Your genes aren't totally in charge of your body: you have a choice about many aspects of the way you live your life, from what you eat to how you exercise. In the following section, we'll consider the factors that influence physical well-being and explore what you can do to trump your genes and live longer.

PART TWO

Physical
Well-being

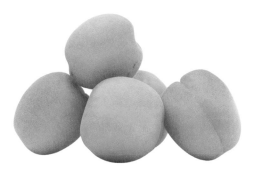

Long living parents
+ **10 YEARS**

It's been recognized for centuries that longevity tends to run in families—if your parents or grandparents lived to a ripe old age, then you stood a better chance of notching up the years, too. It turns out there's a genetic explanation for this.

The Framingham Heart Study found that individuals with long-lived parents had more advantageous cardiovascular risk profiles in middle age compared with those whose parents died younger. They were less likely to smoke or have high blood pressure, and had lower blood cholesterol levels, with a more healthy fat and cholesterol profile.

In a study of Ashkenazi Jews who had passed or nearly reached the century mark, it was found that centenarians tend to have, due to an unusual variation in the ApoC3 gene, a specific genetic profile linked to the healthy storage and breakdown of fats in the body. They are more likely to have lower blood cholesterol levels and less likely to have high blood pressure; they also have greater sensitivity to the hormone insulin, an indication that diabetes is less likely to be a problem. Conversely, centenarians are less likely to carry the unhealthy ApoE4 gene, which promotes the formation of atherosclerosis (the cause of heart disease) at an early age, and more likely to carry the ApoE2 gene, which protects against cardiovascular disease and Alzheimer's.

On a more practical level, those who live to a great age may simply have discovered the right lifestyle formula of nutrition, exercise, and rest, or had the sense to avoid nasty accidents. Watch them and learn!

Only child

5 YEARS? —

If you have lots of brothers and sisters, you probably know what it can be like to grow up in a large family, fighting for attention from tired parents and competing with one another to get enough food at the dinner table. You might think you're missing out on the tranquillity and one-on-one attention a single child enjoys.

Think again—as you get older, the "protective role" of the large family kicks in, and the benefits of having plenty of people around begin to show. Research has found that grandparents who have few siblings live shorter lives than those with lots of siblings; being a single child could mean you lose five years of your life expectancy. If you're a parent, you'll notice a similar effect from having lots of children: they might wear you out when you are a young parent, but in the end they help to keep you going.

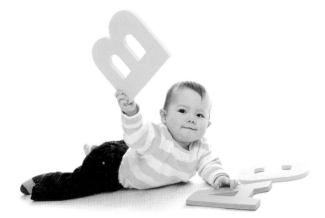

Bad genes
— 10 YEARS

The genes we inherit play a major part in determining how long we live: for instance, a set of rogue genes could knock as much as 10 years off your life. This is because not only do genes influence physical fitness, but they shape our intellectual ability to understand what is necessary to stay healthy. Brain power, common sense, and personality—all strongly influenced by the our genes—affect how we work to afford all those health necessities and fight off disease.

But the main genetic determinants of longevity are those that affect the way the cells maintain and repair themselves. For example, centenarians have higher levels than the general population of a genetic product called PARP-1, a key chemical messenger involved in repair.

How to make the most of your genetic destiny

- Study your family and learn about the genetic influences you are likely to be carrying.

- Take lifestyle steps relevant to your genetics. If you carry genes that leave you with dangerously high cholesterol levels, you must make efforts, from an early age, to control your cholesterol intake and treat the high levels if necessary.

- Make sure you get regular screening for diseases to which you may be vulnerable.

- Follow good medical advice when you do develop disease.

Not only is repair more efficient in the long-lived, but genetic diseases are less likely. People who reach 100 are much less likely to carry genes associated with cancer, disease of the blood vessels, degenerative diseases of the nerves and brain, or diabetes (see entry 21 for more).

The aging process seems to be controlled by telomeres, tiny structures found at the ends of each chromosome (the structures in the cell nucleus that contain the genes). Every time the cell divides, the telomeres are torn a little shorter, like frayed ends. Eventually they become so short that the cell can no longer divide and the tissues cannot be refreshed, so aging changes start to appear.

Scientists in Utah have shown that a person's telomere length, once they reach the age of 60, may be a good indication of their life expectancy. Those with longer telomeres lived on average five years longer than those with short telomeres. People with the shortest telomeres at 60 were three times more likely to get heart disease and nearly twice as likely to die as the others, especially from heart disease and pneumonia.

Anti-aging drug treatments may eventually be developed that lengthen the telomeres. But beware—we already know that telomeres can be lengthened by an enzyme called telomerase, which is particularly found in cancer cells. This may be how cancer cells keep dividing and growing, while at the same time the rest of the body ages.

Genes ultimately account for only 25 percent of what determines longevity. Environment and chance can significantly overrule their powers, and most of us can do something to dodge and weave around the influence of our genes.

Girls rule!

+ **10 YEARS**

In all developed countries and most undeveloped ones, women outlive men, usually by about 10 percent of the average life span. In the USA and northern Europe, women are six times more likely than men to live to 100.

The reason for this difference in life span lies in a complex mix of environmental, genetic, cultural, and anthropological factors. One possible biological factor is the influence of sex hormones. The male hormone testosterone has been associated with increased aggressive and competitive behavior, leading to risks of an early death due to violence, accidents, and risk-taking.

In certain cases, testosterone, especially at supraphysiological levels, can lower HDL ("good" cholesterol) levels. The female hormone estrogen, conversely, increases "good" cholesterol levels. Furthermore, women may have weaker inflammatory activity than men, which, though increasing the risk of serious life-threatening infections, lowers their chance of developing coronary heart disease.

Studies on telomeres (entry 23) also show that men have shorter telomeres than women of the same age—and, therefore, shorter life expectancy.

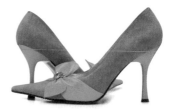

Stay short
5 YEARS

In the 1970s, data gathered from athletes and famous people in the USA showed that shorter, lighter men lived longer than their taller, heavier counterparts. This might have been a backlash to a commonly uttered (but quite untrue) statement that the taller candidate always wins the American Presidential elections (of the 46 elections where heights are known, 54 percent were won by the taller man, 39 percent by the shorter, and in 7 percent they were the same height). The data didn't cause much of a stir—short people already knew that, despite claims that taller people always got the top jobs or glamorous partners, life could be just as sweet closer to the earth.

But then in 1992 the World Health Organization published a report showing that normal male American citizens less than 5 feet 9 inches tall lived nearly five years longer than those over this height. There was no reliable explanation, just a suggestion that taller people burned through calories—and life—faster.

Animal studies also showed that smaller animals within the same species generally lived longer. Since then, all sorts of other research of varying scientific validity has been thrown into the ring to suggest that taller people are more susceptible to damage by pollutants and other chemicals, more likely to develop a variety of cancers, and ultimately more prone to age-related disease.

Obesity

— 3 YEARS

Being fat can be fatal. Countless studies have proven the link between weight and mortality. More acute levels of obesity introduce greater risks of suffering a heart attack or stroke, developing cancer or diabetes, or being afflicted with joint disease. Metabolic syndrome victims—obesity with high blood pressure, diabetes or insulin resistance, and abnormal cholesterol levels—are three times more likely to die earlier than normal for their age.

A 2006 National Institutes of Health study in the US compiled data from more than half a million Americans and found that even small increases in body mass index (BMI—see the next page) can lead to premature death. In middle-aged men and women who had never smoked, simply being overweight (BMI of 25–30) was associated with a 20 to 40 percent increased risk for death. Death rates rise substantially when BMI goes over 30—a morbidly obese person could lose seven years of his or her life.

The key to weight control is healthy eating and regular exercise—it's that simple. You should take steps such as measuring your weight once a week so you can't kid yourself. Find a sensible eating plan you can stick to—and avoid crash diets. Find exercise you enjoy and will keep doing. Make the most of available support, such as slimming groups and counseling. Also talk to your doctor about medical treatments for weight loss.

Being underweight

1 YEAR   —

Being too thin isn't healthy either: studies have found that the risk of death rises as BMI drops below 24.5. In fact, according to the Institute of Preventative Medicine in Copenhagen, curvy is best. Their studies found that women with wide hips were 87 percent less likely to die from heart disease than slim-hipped women. Fat in that area contains a natural anti-inflammatory chemical called adiponectin, which keeps arteries healthy; women with hips less than 40 inches wide don't get this protection.

How to measure your body mass index

The body mass index (BMI) measure

Find your height in inches and square the figure. Divide your weight in pounds by your height squared, and multiply by 703. A normal BMI is between 18.5 and 25. A BMI above 30 indicates that you are obese and is associated with a greater risk of death. Note, though, that BMI doesn't distinguish between the weight of fat and that of muscle, so fit, muscular athletes may be misclassified.

Your waist circumference

Waist circumference is now thought to be a better indicator of body fat and risk than BMI. A circumference of more than 32 inches for women and 37 inches for men increases the risk of cardiovascular diseases and diabetes.

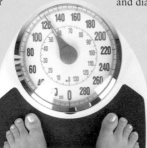

Eating less

+ # 1 YEAR?

There is no doubt that what we eat and drink play a vital part in keeping us healthy and therefore staying the course for the life span that humans can normally expect (perhaps as many as 120 years). Experiments in dietary restriction since the 1930s have shown that restricting calorie intake extends life in a wide variety of creatures, including rats and nearly every invertebrate studied, such as worms and flies. But what about humans?

The facts are these: during normal aging, a progressive state of inflammation builds in the body, especially in the nervous system and brain. Meanwhile, dietary restriction is known to reduce the amount of inflammation in the body, and seems to increase the brain's ability to repair itself. If the theory of dietary restriction holds, eating less often or fasting temporarily may eventually point to an extension of life: we may gain a year in life for every two years spent on a 1,000- to 1,500-calorie diet. For now, though, this strategy is unproven for humans.

You could try cutting down on calories or eating less frequently, but don't go overboard: a drastic reduction in calories and nutrients could damage the body, leaving your immune system shaky and vulnerable to infections and many other conditions.

Don't try sniffing at food to calm your appetite! Not only will it make you feel more hungry, but research on Drosophila fruit flies (which, strangely, age like humans) shows that simply the smell of food can significantly reverse the life-prolonging effects of calorie restriction.

Food obsessions

5 YEARS? —

Researching longer-living people, scientists (or at least some crafty marketing people) heard of a tribe in the remote Himalayan mountains called the Hunzas, which included an unusually large number of people living way past 100. This longevity was attributed to the humble apricot. Cut off from the rest of the world in a valley ringed by high mountains, the Hunzas were, until recently, forced to survive on a meager diet of apricots, walnuts, buckwheat cakes, and an awful lot of vegetables. The Hunzas eat apricots by the handful, drink the juice, smear the flesh on their skin, and even burn the kernels for fuel—and rarely suffer common Western health problems such as cancer or heart disease.

But while scientists acknowledge that apricots contain high levels of carotenoids, a natural type of antioxidant (see entry 33), researchers also credit the low-stress lifestyle, the endless physical toil, and the primitive, caveman-style diet of the Hunzas.

The low-fat content of the Hunzas' already restricted diet keeps daily calorie intake down, too. Such restricted intake has been noted in other communities with a reputation for long life, such as in Okinawa in Japan, where people survive on 20 percent fewer calories than the national average. Dietary restriction is a key area in aging research (see entry 28). But this doesn't mean restricting yourself to obsessively eating just one food—doing so will make you miss out on vital nutrients, and could eventually take five years off your life.

Vitamins

+ 3 YEARS

The need for vitamins has been recognized for centuries—the ancient Egyptians knew that eating liver could prevent night blindness (now known to be due to vitamin A deficiency), and lemons and limes were first used by the British Royal Navy in the eighteenth century to prevent scurvy (a disease caused by vitamin C deficiency).

We know that vitamins are required in minute amounts in our diet for essential metabolic processes within the body, and that they are vital for health—without them life may be shortened by disease. But scientific research has as yet been unable to determine if taking extra vitamins could offer particular health benefits or prolong life.

Governmental guidelines suggest the amount of each vitamin that you should get in your diet every day, and eating a good balance of foods should ensure that you get adequate amounts of the vitamins you need. But some people argue that these recommended allowances are simply a measure of what is enough to keep at bay those conditions recognized to be the result of vitamin deficiencies, rather than proposing an amount to actively promote health in other ways—by improving the immune system, for example. As many studies have conflicting findings, the evidence isn't yet clear that higher levels of many vitamins can definitively prolong the human life span. Stay on top of the most recent RDA recommendations and discuss taking additional supplements with your doctor.

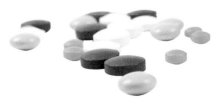

Fiber

1 YEAR +

Fiber helps keep you regular, but can it help you live longer? Unfortunately, research has not been definitively convincing. Fiber is particularly recommended as a protection against cardiovascular disease and cancer, but tests involving a high-fiber diet have produced varying results, either suggesting an insignificant reduction in death from any cause, including heart disease, or proposing a 28 percent reduction in the likelihood of developing heart failure.

The case against cancer is stronger, however, as animal experiments show a reduction in colon cancer. Surveys of people who eat a lot of fiber suggest that this works for humans, too, although trials where fiber has been specifically added to the diet to prevent cancer haven't shown an effect. Meanwhile, one new study has shown that fiber from cereals and fruit may protect against breast cancer.

Although the real value of this much-lauded element of our diet isn't clear, it's best, for now, to keep going for the grain: a long-term, high-fiber diet could well turn out to add a year or more to your life.

How to add necessary fiber to your diet

- Eat soluble fiber, found in legumes, fruit, and vegetables. It lowers cholesterol levels, helps delay absorption of foods, and aids blood sugar control.

- Eat insoluble fiber, from wholegrain cereals, fruit, and vegetables. It improves bowel function.

Too much sugar

— **1 YEAR?**

For any dentist, the link between sugar consumption and mortality is clear: sugar in the diet leads to dental cavities, which leads to losing your teeth; this leads, in turn, to a reduced ability to eat healthy food, and ultimately pushes you toward an early grave. This might have been true before the days of modern dentistry and fluoride toothpaste (or true for those who, sadly, can't afford modern dentistry), but today most of us manage to avoid tooth decay and keep our teeth despite a sugary diet.

If you brush regularly and go for dental check-ups as you should, is there any reason why you should cut down on sugar?

Low sugar intake can help to control weight and reduce the risks associated with obesity. Furthermore, eating less sugar or sugary foods—and keeping a wary eye out for refined sugar, in particular—may be an important part of the dietary-restriction strategy for improving health and prolonging life (see entry 28).

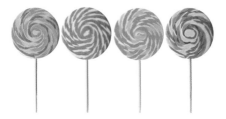

Antioxidants

2 YEARS +

One of the main theories about why the body degenerates as we age is based on a chemical process called oxidation. During normal metabolism the body produces unstable molecules called free radicals. Other factors in the environment around us also increase free radical production (see entry 61). Free radicals cause oxidation— this is dangerous as it damages the body's cells and tissues, and has been implicated in all the major killer diseases.

Fortunately, we have a supply of natural antidotes called antioxidants, which mop up free radicals. But levels of antioxidants fall as we age, leading to increasing damage to cells and tissues. By increasing our intake of antioxidants as we get older (or avoiding free-radical-producing pollutants), we may be able to protect ourselves from this process.

A wide range of chemicals found in different foods can act as antioxidants but some of the most important are beta-carotene and the antioxidant vitamins A, C, and E. As far as antioxidant supplements go, however, studies have been disappointing. Some trials found only minimal and inconsistent evidence that any single vitamin supplement, combined antioxidant supplement, or multivitamin combination has a significant benefit in cardiovascular disease, while others found that beta-carotene used to prevent cancer might even increase the risk of death from other causes. Research on people who follow a diet rich in antioxidants, rather than relying on supplements, however, has been promising, for example in reducing the risk of Alzheimer's disease. Something in the chemical complexity of food could be key here. The best advice for now is simply to keep your diet healthy and wait for further results about supplements.

Fast food

— **4 YEARS**

Manufacturers face considerable challenges to prepare foods that will taste good, have a reasonable shelf life, and return a good profit. To manage this they pack foods with preservatives, refined sugar, and hydrogenated or trans fats—ingredients that would make a nutritionist shriek.

And for good reason: in experiments, monkeys fed a fast-food diet rich in trans fats grew fatter around the waist than those fed a diet containing the same number of calories overall while being rich in unsaturated fats. The monkeys on the fast-food diet also developed signs of insulin resistance, an early indicator of diabetes. After six years the trans-fat monkeys were 7.2 percent heavier than before (compared to a 1.2 percent weight gain in the other group), and had 30 percent more fat in their abdomen, which is particularly linked to heart disease. If you regularly eat fast foods or pre-packaged foods, you could lose four years off your life span.

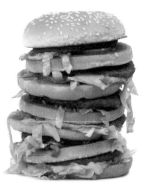

Mediterranean diet

5 YEARS +

It's not just the sun and sea they're blessed with. Scientific research has shown that people who live in the Mediterranean are the best candidates for longevity and also enjoy low rates of heart disease. Their life-prolonging diet is linked to a lower death rate from all sorts of diseases, including heart disease, and may also lower the risk of Alzheimer's by as much as 40 percent.

Key to this diet is the generous amount of fruit, vegetables, and nuts consumed, and the lack of processed foods. Increasing fruit and vegetables from two to five portions a day can greatly reduce the risk of many cancers, while it's known that a vegetarian diet is linked to a premature death rate 20 percent lower than for meat eaters.

But it's the whole lifestyle that counts: also central to this culture are two other factors you can't ignore—more physical activity and an extended social support system.

What to have in your kitchen

Although there is great diversity between Mediterranean countries, common dietary threads include large amounts of fruit, vegetables, beans, nuts, cereals, and seeds; olive oil, fish, and poultry to be consumed in moderation; a little red meat and dairy produce; and wine, but again to be taken in moderate amounts.

Good fats

+ **1 YEAR**

Fat is an important part of our diet but if you want to avoid the No. 1 killer in the Western world—heart disease—you need to choose your fats carefully. Some dietary fats are much healthier than others; in fact, making sure to include healthy fats in your diet could earn you an extra year in your normal life expectancy.

When you think about fat in your diet, the aim should be to control the overall amount you consume (it's recommended that no more than 11% of calories each day should come from fats) and, more specifically, keep down levels of LDL-cholesterol, which is one of the worst criminals in cardiovascular disease. Saturated fat, trans-fatty acids (TFAs), and cholesterol in the diet all increase the risk of cardiovascular disease. TFAs may also raise levels of LDL-cholesterol ("bad" cholesterol) and lower levels of HDL-cholesterol ("good" cholesterol). But mono- and polyunsaturated fats don't seem to have this harmful profile and may even help lower LDL-cholesterol slightly. How far eating the right fats will help you live longer is still being tested, but there is some evidence that it reduces heart problems and early death, so there is no harm in changing your habits for the better.

The main types of fat in food include saturated fat, which is found mostly in foods from animals and some plants, for instance butter, cream, milk, cheeses, coconut oil, and palm oil. Mono- and polyunsaturated fat are found mainly in fish (such as salmon and trout) and also in seeds, avocados and plant oils (for instance olive oil and sunflower oil). Trans fats (also known as trans-fatty acids or TFAs) occur in small amounts in various animal products, and are formed when vegetable oils are put through the hydrogenation process to make margarine, shortening, and cooking oils for use in processed foods such as biscuits, fried foods, and cakes. TFAs are used by manufacturers as they allow foods to have a long shelf life and give food desirable shape, taste, and texture.

To reduce total, saturated, and TFA fats, use low-fat versions of dairy products (such as semi-skimmed or skimmed milk), buy lean cuts of meat and remove visible fat and skin from the meat before you cook it, and use less fat in cooking (grill and bake rather than fry or roast). Choose small amounts of fats and oils that are rich in monounsaturates (e.g. olive oil) or polyunsaturates (e.g. sunflower oil) rather than saturated fats such as butter.

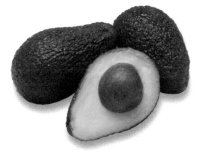

How to get the right fat in your diet

- Keep in mind the advice from the American Heart Association:

- Fat should account for less than 25 to 35 percent of your total calorie intake each day.

- Most fat in your diet should be unsaturated.

- Less than 7 percent of calories should be from saturated fat.

- Less than 1 percent of calories should be from trans fats.

- You should limit your cholesterol intake to less than 300 milligrams per day (less than 200 milligrams per day if you have heart disease).

- Beware the fat hidden in packaged and processed foods—always check labels. Avoid trans fats, and remember that unhydrogenated vegetable oils are better than hydrogenated ones.

- Choose soft margarine instead of hard margarine or butter.

Minerals

✚ **3 YEARS**

Besides playing various vital roles in the healthy functioning of your body, minerals keep the immune system working well. As we get older, however, we are more likely to become deficient in certain minerals because of poor diet, increasing needs, or excess loss from the body. Mineral deficiency may play a part in many life-shortening diseases. For example, people with a lower magnesium intake are more likely to develop Type 2 (non-insulin dependent) diabetes while low levels of selenium are linked to poor immune function and an increased risk of cancer.

Magic minerals include calcium for good bones, iron to transport oxygen in the blood, selenium to make certain enzymes, magnesium to help important biochemical reactions in the body, and zinc to slow age-related deterioration of cells.

There are various ways in which we can increase our intake of minerals. Start by eating a wide variety of foods, as different minerals are found in different foods. For example you could get calcium from dairy products, and fish such as salmon and sardines; iron from red meat, eggs, beans, and leafy green vegetables; and zinc from meat and legumes. Though it is important to note that modern farming and food preparation can deplete levels of certain minerals. For example, chromium and selenium levels may be higher in organic foods. Another way of adding minerals to your diet is to take a daily supplement if you or your doctor think you need it. Older people, especially postmenopausal women, may particularly benefit from calcium supplements, for example, to keep their bones strong.

Omega-3s

5 YEARS +

Truly nature's own wonder workers, Omega-3s, an important group of polyunsaturated fatty acids (PUFAs), are essential for growth and development. They do a fantastic job of preventing coronary heart disease, high blood pressure, diabetes, and arthritis, among a host of other conditions.

Humans evolved on a diet that contained roughly equal amounts of Omega-3 and Omega-6 fatty acids. But this balance has gone out of kilter in the last couple of centuries: we now consume as much as 20 or 30 times more Omega-6s than Omega-3s, partly because of the increased amount of certain vegetable oils in our diet. This shifts the physiology of the body to a state where blood is thicker, blood vessels are more likely to go into spasm, and clots are more likely to form. Although Omega-3s counteract this effect, reducing inflammation and thrombosis, we are generally not getting enough for them to do the job right.

But there are ways in which we can up our Omega-3 intake. Oily fish such as mackerel, salmon or sardines are a good source and you should aim to eat at least two portions a week. Replace sunflower, safflower, sesame, and corn oils with flaxseed, walnut, and canola oils, which are richer in Omega-3 alpha-linolenic acid. And consider supplements after consulting with your doctor—they may be the only way to get enough Omega-3s.

Bad posture
— 2 YEARS

Stop! Don't move—think about how your spine is shaped right now. Are you slumped over your desk? Uncomfortably perched on a chair? Is your pelvis crooked or twisted around your spine? If so, you could be putting your health at risk and chipping years off your life expectancy.

Now, sit upright. Plant your feet squarely on the floor and let your shoulders relax. Take some deep breaths. In these three short steps, you've taken positive action toward living a longer and healthier life. Doesn't that feel better? The body is a finely tuned piece of structural engineering. In order to work and move healthily, it needs to be fully aligned. A body out of line puts abnormal strain on the muscles, tendons, and ligaments, wearing out the joints, bones, and muscles, and perhaps affecting the internal organs as well. Poor posture leads to lower back pain and arthritis, among other back and spinal injuries.

The links with longevity are plenty. Lower back pain frequently interferes with work, leading to a poorer quality of life and poorer general health, while older people with humped back (hyperkyphosis) have been shown to be more likely to die earlier, especially due to cardiovascular disease.

You can improve your posture at work by making sure your desk or work area is ergonomically designed. And get the advice of a licensed back specialist, who can advise you on exercises to align your bones and muscles. It's all about strengthening the muscles of your back and abdomen to hold your spine straight: help yourself by asking a gym trainer for a special program, or take up yoga.

Stretching

1 YEAR   +

Limbs that are stiff and tight are more prone to injury, and put abnormal strain on other areas of the body, leading to back pain, arthritis, and other problems. A lack of suppleness can cause tightness of the hamstring muscles in the leg, for example, which is often a major factor in back pain and knee conditions.

Flexibility protects the muscles and joints from injury, reducing the risks of torn muscle fibers (strains) and torn ligaments (sprains). It helps to make exercise easier, allowing the musculoskeletal system to develop stamina and become strong. Flexibility also helps to maintain balance and reduces the risk of falls (see entry 43). There's a very important feel-good factor about being supple and lithe, too. Movement doesn't seem to be such a struggle. Bending, stretching, and shaking become effortless, and you want to get out there and dance (or run, jump, or play tennis—whatever you like).

How to get flexible

- Stretch each muscle group for 15–30 seconds every day to increase your range of movement.

- Stretch until you feel a slight pulling but not pain. Hold the stretch here. As the muscle relaxes, increase the stretch until it pulls again. Be sure not to "bounce" during a stretch, because this risks injury.

- Try an exercise that specifically involves stretching, such as yoga or Pilates.

Getting active

+ 4 YEARS

Exercise can reduce the risk of heart disease, diabetes, colon cancer, and breast cancer, and generally keep death at bay. The Harvard Alumni Study, carried out over 38 years, concluded that a brisk, hour-long walk five days a week nearly halves the risk of having a stroke. Even walking for half an hour a day five times a week drops the risk by 24 percent. Other research shows that just 30 minutes of exercise a day cuts the risk of breast cancer by half for postmenopausal women. Exercise sparks brain cells into action, too: walking (or dancing or swimming—the choice is yours) for just 45 minutes three times a week helps reverse the natural decline of your IQ.

Think you're too late to start? The Harvard study showed that people over 75 who took up exercise and quit smoking could add, on average, almost two years to their lives. And before you yell "I haven't got the time!" remember that something is better than nothing. You can break up your exercise into small chunks—half a mile here, a third of a mile there—as what matters is the daily total. Among those Harvard alumni who had no major health risk factors, a weekend-warrior approach to exercise (that is, just one to two episodes a week, generating a total of 1,000 calories) was enough to postpone mortality.

As American health motivator Robert Sweetgall says, "Get off your ass and start moving around!"

Over-exercising
2 YEARS?

In the 1970s and '80s, dance fitness suddenly threatened to take over the exercise world—remember the arrival of big hair, Lycra, and Irene Cara leaping across the screen in Fame? We were urged to "go for the burn"—to exercise so fast and so furiously that the muscles didn't have time to get the oxygen they needed, and so had to switch to anaerobic work. As a result, a chemical called lactic acid built up in the muscles, leaving a burning sensation that was unpleasantly firey (or nicely hot, if this was your sort of thing). The muscles also burned up lots of calories during this time—another meaning for the term "burn."

These days, scientists wonder if regularly going for the burn could actually lead to an early grave. Going for the burn is exhausting and, although some find it a buzz, it can be so unpleasant that it puts you off exercise for good. It's also far more likely to lead to injury.

You don't have to go crazy to keep fit; there are dozens of activities to choose from. For example, walking, especially walking uphill, is just as good an exercise as running. Sometimes it's best to go slow and steady—the way of the tortoise rather than the hare.

Good balance

+ 3 YEARS

In China and other Eastern countries you often see elderly people out early in the morning gently practicing tai chi in the local park. They are doing their best to avoid an event responsible for more deaths in older people in the Western world than anything else—a fall.

Human beings are inherently unstable creatures. Walking on two legs we have a narrow base and a high center of gravity. To move without tumbling over, we normally rely on complex mechanisms that detect our state of balance and rapidly correct wobbles. While young we can lean, stumble, or trip and still finish upright. If we do fall, the worst result may be a fractured wrist, and this is a break that doesn't make much difference to life span. As we get older those mechanisms are increasingly likely to fail, and the chance increases of our ending up flat on the floor, even after the slightest challenge to our balance. Once you're over 65, you have a one in three chance of falling each year. With a loss of the necessary protective mechanisms, a fall can often result in a broken hip or a fractured skull. As the person is often left lying alone and with help beyond reach for hours, problems such as pneumonia, hypothermia, or dehydration may set in.

To reduce your chances of an early death by falling, you should follow a simple program of muscle strengthening and balance retraining. Take a tip from the East— refining your balance through exercises like tai chi can halve the risk of a fall.

Couch potato
8 YEARS ▬

According to the Stanford School of Medicine, life on the sofa is life on the edge. Inactivity is now considered an independent risk factor for a shorter life, along with smoking, high blood pressure, and high cholesterol. Lying around on the sofa makes you more prone to heart disease, diabetes, back pain, and falls and accidents when you do eventually drag yourself to your feet.

The Stanford study showed that every increase in exercise capacity made the risk of death from any cause drop by 12 percent. Don't confuse this with over-exercising, though (see entry 42): the most effective way to build exercise capacity is by slow, steady increases in training.

And any little bit you do helps. A British Regional Heart Study showed that, while vigorous activity halves the risk of death, any activity is better than none.

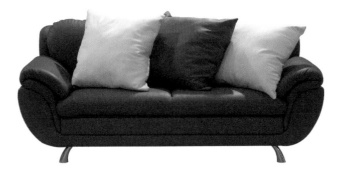

Not getting enough sleep
— **5 YEARS**

Good-quality sleep can be positively linked to successful aging and longer survival, while disruptive sleep patterns tend to be a sign of faster aging and disease. Sleep studies have shown that fragmented sleep raises levels of blood fats, cholesterol, cortisol, and blood pressure—all powerful risk factors for cardiovascular disease. Furthermore, lack of sleep reduces brain power and vigilance, leaving sleepy people prone to accidents during the day.

Some studies even suggest that sleep may be the most important predictor of how long you will live—more important, even, than your cholesterol level or blood pressure reading. A large study in the 1950s by the American Cancer Society found that the highest death rates were among those people who said that they slept for just four hours or fewer a night. Those who slept excessively—nine to 10 or more hours a night—had higher death rates as well. More recent research has confirmed these findings, with those people sleeping six to seven hours a night living the longest.

How to get better sleep

- Stick to a regular sleep schedule, with the same bedtime every night, and a regular relaxing routine to help you wind down.

- Avoid late-night stimulants such as coffee (even decaffeinated), tea, hot chocolate, and alcohol. Try herbal teas, especially camomile, or milk instead.

- If you can't get to sleep in 20 minutes in bed, get up and sit quietly for a while before trying again. Don't watch TV or put on bright lights as this will tell your brain it's time to wake up.

Napping during the day
1 YEAR +

People living in the tropics traditionally take a siesta or short nap after lunch. It's a logical way to escape the intense heat of the midday sun, which can put strain on the body, raising blood pressure and heart rate. But are daytime naps really good for you? It's a subject of great debate.

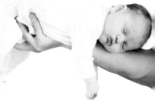

A study from Greece showed that regular midday naps of about 30 minutes may help reduce the risk of heart disease, especially in men, possibly because they help to break the tension of the day and relieve stress. In the study people who napped at least three times a week for almost 30 minutes had a 37 percent reduction in the risk of dying from a heart attack or another heart-related problem.

A longer nap can disrupt your daily sleep pattern, however, and alter the quality of sleep at night. It may also be a sign that night time sleep is inadequate, for example because of potentially fatal conditions such as obstructive sleep apnea. If you find you need more substantial snoozes during the day, it may be time to get your health checked out.

Yoga

✚ 5 YEARS?

According to yoga philosophy, it's the flexibility of the spine, not the number of years, that determines a person's age. Yoga slows down the aging process by giving elasticity to the spine, firming up the skin, removing stress from the body, strengthening the abdominal muscles, and correcting poor posture. The deep rhythmic breathing in yoga relieves respiratory complaints including asthma, while the increased oxygen boosts muscle strength.

Yoga is said to affect all the important determinants of a long life—the brain, spine, internal organs, and circulation—and to have a marked effect on pituitary, thyroid, adrenal, and sex glands. This produces a feeling of well-being and extends sexual virility well into old age. Yoga claims that inverted postures can help to prevent gray hair (due to increased blood supply to the hair follicles) and facial wrinkles, while increased pressure on neck muscles means that vision and hearing can be improved, too.

What is certainly true is that the relaxation techniques and physical exercise involved in yoga result in a positive mental and emotional state, making you feel more energized, relaxed, and generally optimistic.

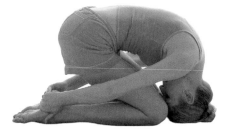

Good dental hygiene
6 YEARS +

Good dental care could actually help you live longer by preventing other common killers, according to the American Academy of Periodontology. Our mouths are full of bacteria that may be harmful if they get into the bloodstream. Healthy gums help form a barrier that the bacteria cannot cross, but if we don't look after our gums an infection known as periodontal disease can set in, breaking down the defenses and allowing the bacteria an easy route to enter the body. Recent research has linked periodontal infections to heart disease, diabetes, and respiratory disease. Unfortunately, too, the risk of periodontal disease increases as we get older, raising the general level of inflammation in the body (see entry 28 for why this might be important).

Remember to take care of your teeth and gums by brushing frequently and thoroughly, flossing properly, and seeing your dentist regularly. He or she will also be able to spot if you develop cancer of the mouth or oral cavity.

Good sex

+ **4 YEARS**

Shocking news! Sex is good for you! Research shows that the more often men experience orgasms, the lower their risk of dying. Those who have frequent orgasms (at least twice a week) are half as likely to die than those who don't, from all causes but especially heart disease. There's also evidence that men who ejaculate frequently are less likely to develop cancer of the prostate.

Some early research into sex and health has suggested that while frequency of sex is associated with mortality in men—the Swedes discovered, for example, that once men give up having sex they are more likely to die—it is the enjoyment of sex, rather, that is linked to death rates in women. Studies have found that women who don't enjoy a fulfilling sex life because their partner has problems with premature ejaculation or impotence, are more likely to have a heart attack.

The available research doesn't really tell us enough yet, but it certainly overturns the old-fashioned view in some communities that sex drains vigor and wellbeing. It also backs up the common belief that what matters a lot for men is how often they have sex—the physical activity may be most important—but for women the quality of the emotional experience may have greater value. Simply being close, kissing, and enjoying loving tenderness may do more for a woman's health than the physical workout of hot passion. For the same reason, "bad" sex (that is, when her partner is cold and insensitive, or simply when she is worried that he isn't enjoying the experience) is more likely to be detrimental to her well-being.

It is easy to imagine how good sex, especially within a stable relationship, may be good for your health: intimacy, comfort, and pleasure all relieve stress and bring happiness, while the physical effort gives the cardiovascular system a good workout. So get it while you can!

Risky sex

8 YEARS

We've found that sex is good for you—so why ruin its positive effects by catching a sexually transmitted disease (STD), especially one such as HIV, which could kill you?

The number of people living with HIV in the world has increased considerably and continues to rise. If you have unprotected sex, you will be at risk from sexually transmitted infections such as HIV. The risk is even greater if you have frequent, casual partners.

While ever-improving medical treatments mean that HIV isn't the death sentence it once was, it still can't be cured. Modern treatments can keep the virus under control and limit the damage that it does, but they can have troublesome side effects and the virus may become resistant.

HIV isn't the only STD that you need to protect yourself from. Other potentially fatal viral infections such as hepatitis B and hepatitis C may be passed on during sex, with serious implications for long term health. As many as 70 percent of people with hepatitis C, for example, will develop chronic liver disease and up to 5 percent will die as a result.

And while syphilis, gonorrhoea, chlamydia, warts, and herpes may be treatable, they can cause major health problems, affecting hopes for a long and happy life in other ways. The most common bacterial cause of STDs, chlamydia, is often carried unwittingly by men and women who are symptomless and unaware that they are passing it on. Silently chlamydia may wreak its damage—among women it is a common cause of inflammation in the pelvis, leading to chronic pelvic pain and a high risk of infertility.

Intelligence

+ 2 YEARS

You don't have to be a genius to figure out that being clever could help you live longer. Intelligent people are more likely to know what to do to keep healthy, access precious resources (including healthcare), and fight for the best treatment.

This may purely be a matter of wealth—people with higher IQs tend to get better-paid jobs and can afford a healthier lifestyle and better medical treatment. If you are born into poverty or difficult social circumstances, it's hard to break free from the stresses of life, no matter how smart you are. But perhaps the most important underlying factor is smoking. The Scottish Mental Health Survey found that children with a lower IQ had a higher risk of dying from lung and stomach cancer, as well as cardiovascular disease, mostly because they are more likely to smoke as adults.

According to researchers at the London School of Economics, IQ is particularly important in dealing with the hazards of modern life. Using data from the World Bank and the United Nations, they found that in developed countries, IQ was seven to eight times more strongly related to life expectancy than income was. But in primitive societies without modern hazards, wealth was far more relevant.

So if you live in the modern world, do everything you can to nurture your brain. And if you just can't pump up your IQ then find someone intelligent as a life partner to boost your chances!

Being informed
2 YEARS

+

When it comes to looking after your body and doing what you need to do to prevent premature aging, information is, undoubtedly, power. Ignorance is a fast track to illness and an early death. But an understanding of the particular health issues you face as you grow older will help to keep your engine running smoothly and allow you to spot the first signs of trouble. You also need to know how to separate the truth from the hype and to learn what doesn't work so that you don't waste your hard-earned cash on worthless anti-aging pills and potions.

Do you know what your cholesterol level should be and what it actually is? When was the last time you thought about your blood pressure? And do you know what screening you should be going for and how often? Just a few of the many questions that you need answers to if you want to live forever. You're reading this book, so you're already on the right path!

How to be informed about your health

Take power into your own hands and ask yourself these basic questions:

- What are your cholesterol and blood pressure levels? What should they be? If they are high, what are you doing to bring them down?

- Based on your age and family health history, what health screenings should you regularly schedule?

- What health risks do you personally face—from your genes, your job, or your habits?

Bad doctor

— **4 YEARS**

If you want to live forever, you're going to need your own personal health expert. A good doctor should understand your particular medical history and social issues, and should be able to schedule you for the necessary vaccinations or recommend routine screening programs that may help to prevent cancer of the breast, colon, or cancer.

You need to have a good working relationship with your doctor so that you are comfortable asking about anything you need to know, without feeling embarrassed or as if you are wasting his or her time. If you don't like your doctor or don't get along well with them, it may be time to think about seeing someone else. Your doctor won't mind—we all understand that people relate in many different ways and we can't all get along with everybody else.

One of the best ways to find a good doctor is to ask your friends for a recommendation. And don't wait until you are ill to start looking—living longer is all about prevention of disease, not just fire-fighting illness. Before you make your decision, it is also a good idea to check the doctor's qualifications and special interests such as women's health or cardiology, to see if they match your likely needs or current conditions.

Once you have registered with a practice, when you meet your doctor, be honest with him or her—this is not the time to be shy or coy about health issues that may trouble you, however trivial you might think they are. It is also important that if you don't get along, you get out—and find someone else.

Frequent pregnancies
6 MONTHS?   —

Not so long ago, pregnancy could be clearly linked to a higher chance of an early death as it brought about significant risks. Modern healthcare in developed countries has greatly reduced those risks and a woman's chances of dying during pregnancy or childbirth are only about one in 10,000—but these chances do exist. Some of these deaths are as a direct result of the pregnancy, while others occur because pregnancy puts an extra strain on existing health problems. Every pregnancy that goes to full term could bring with it a six-month decrease in life span.

One of the leading causes of maternal death is thrombo-embolic disease, or the formation of clots. Eclampsia (where the blood pressure becomes very high), haemorrhage, and infections are the other major problems. Because of complications of pregnancy and childbirth, some women are left with serious ill health or disability as well.

Women worried about the risks of pregnancy should give some thought to the amount of time they leave between each pregnancy. Research has shown that when the interval between pregnancies is less than six months, there is an increased risk of bleeding, premature rupture of membranes, infection, anaemia, and death, while an interval longer than 59 months is linked to an increased risk of pre-eclampsia and eclampsia.

With all the risks taken into account, however, you'll see that there are myriad benefits from living together as a family, including blissfully happy moments that, even if they don't extend life, certainly add to its quality (see Part One).

Hormone replacement

+ **1 YEAR?**

Levels of many hormones in the body fall with age. As these hormone levels fall and symptoms of disease appear, there is a clear justification for trying to replenish those failing hormones. But the scientific evidence to prove the benefits of

Hormone help

Levels of many hormones in the body decrease with age.

- Levels of the female sex hormones estrogen and progesterone drop during menopause. The genital tissues thin, increasing the risk of urinary tract infection, while the risk of osteoporosis and heart disease increase.

- Quantities of growth hormone (GH) and testosterone are diminished, which may result in a decrease in lean body mass and an increase in adipose tissue.

- The pancreas becomes less efficient at producing the hormone insulin, which can lead to diabetes.

- Levels of dehydroepiandrosterone (DHEA), a hormone that is produced by the adrenal gland and is the main precursor of the sex hormones, fall steadily.

- Levels of thyroid hormones can wane, leading to problems such as tiredness, depression, constipation, and dryness of the skin and hair.

- Levels of melatonin may decline, disrupting control of normal body rhythms and resulting in possibly a deterioration of immunity.

hormone replacement therapy (HRT) is controversial. From the 1990s on, many wide-ranging studies have been carried out looking at replacing female sex hormones for women going through menopause; the evidence remains inconclusive—even directly contradictory, in some cases—on how effective HRT actually is and the debate continues.

The evidence for any other type of HRT is also unclear. There have only been small studies of healthy older adults taking human growth hormone, for example, and these found that while injections may increase muscle mass and reduce body fat, they don't actually increase strength: strength training is a cheaper and more effective way to achieve this. Neither is it clear whether human growth hormone can provide other benefits to healthy adults, such as increased bone density and improved mood. Side effects are also a problem, so beware the sales hype. Research has also recently blown apart the claims for DHEA supplements, showing that although they caused hormone levels to rise in the body this did not lead to significant improvements in health or quality of life. Similarly, the positive benefits of melatonin supplements have yet to be proven.

Levels of testosterone in women drop gradually with age, but the levels decline more substantially after a hysterectomy and oophorectomy. Many unapproved supplements are available. At this time, HRT is used in the form of one or more female hormones of estrogen and progesterone for menopausal symptoms, or severe hot flashes. Make sure to get expert advice relevant to your health problem first, before starting any hormone supplements.

Take a look around you. The room you're in, the air you breathe, the weather outside, and the unseen radioactive rays that penetrate your home could all influence whether you will live forever—or at least for a good, long time. Studies of twins—a standard way of looking at the influence of our genes—show that only about 25 percent of the variation in human life span in developed countries is the result of inherited factors. That means that the greatest influence by far on how long we live is what happens to us during our life. One of the most important aspects of this is the environment we live in, and the risks it exposes us to.

The environmental risk factors for disease have changed dramatically in the past couple of hundred years, and you are likely to be exposed to very different dangers than the ones your grandparents or great-grandparents faced. While medieval plumbing systems (or the lack thereof) and the Black Death may not be foremost in your mind, you surely are aware of new environmental risks from chemicals and pollution that have emerged in our post-industrial era.

In this section, we'll take a look at the aging factors in the world in which we live, and how they affect our time on earth.

PART THREE

Environment

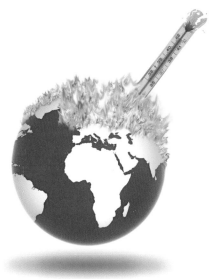

Place of birth

+ **10 YEARS**

Where you were born pulls together a number of factors that can influence how long you might expect to live. If you were born in a developed nation or into a wealthy family in a developing nation, it could make a difference of 10 years in your life span. What makes things more complicated is that even if you eventually move, you still carry the legacy of your birthright with you. The various factors that your birthplace dictates may include:

- **Your genetics:** There are huge regional variations in genetics, with many genetic diseases being particularly prevalent in certain areas. Sickle cell disease, for example, is much more common among people in Africa or of African origin, while gene mutations for cystic fibrosis are more likely to be found in the north of England.
- **Your diet:** Dietary habits are formed early in life and can be hard to change. Children growing up in a fast-food culture are more likely to eat such food, and suffer all its unhealthy effects, for the rest of their life. Conversely, a healthy diet in childhood may protect against disease later in life. Research shows that Asians living in their native country have far lower breast cancer rates than Americans, probably because of a diet rich in vegetables, including soybeans. If those Asians move, as adults, to the USA, the cancer rate goes up just a small amount. But US-born children of Asian immigrants have a 60 percent higher risk of breast cancer. Either a protective factor in the Asian diet in childhood has been lost, or there is a harmful dietary factor at work in the Western diet.
- **Cultural attitudes to health:** In most societies, there are myths and misconceptions about health. These are often passed from generation to

generation and it can be difficult to persuade someone to change their view as they get older. Cultural views on the roles of men and women, for example, also influence longevity. How your parents or grandparents taught you to behave— whether smoking was acceptable, or whether vaccination was considered the devil's magic—may stay with you for life.

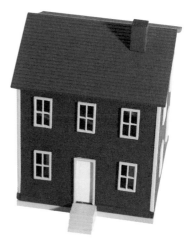

- **Your schooling:** Where you are born is likely to be where you spend your childhood and so where you go to school— that is, if you go to school. Education directly links to longevity (see Fac. 20) because the more you learn, the more healthy and wealthy you are likely to be.
- **Damage done by childhood illness:** From the moment of conception and throughout childhood we are influenced by the environment around us, through war, accidents, disease, and pollution. The effects of childhood illness may be carried with you through later life.

While you can escape most (but not all) of these, the effect they have on your body, your psyche, or your habits in young life may leave a permanent mark on your health and mortality.

City life

— 3 YEARS

"Better beans and bacon in peace than cakes and ale in fear," says the country mouse in Aesop's fable. The town mouse had scoffed at his country cousin's basic diet and taken him to feast in the town. But, chased by large dogs and stressed by urban living, the country mouse soon retreated home.

Both urban and rural life have advantages for health but in general, the more urbanized a nation, the higher the average life expectancy. Development of cities and towns tends to reflect industry, wealth, good communications, and an established social support system. However, within many cities there are areas of intense deprivation where segregated groups live in substandard housing while battling typical urban problems such as traffic pollution and a lack of green space.

So although living in an urbanized nation may help you to live longer, it may be better, if you can afford it, to choose the more rural areas within that nation. If you have to live in a town or city, having walkable green space nearby—and using it—has been shown to be associated with living longer.

The opposite is true for a non-developed nation. Here, city dwelling represents opportunity, wealth, and a longer life (as long as you manage to live in the nice part of town). Life expectancy data from the United Nations shows remarkable similarities between urban slums and rural areas in low-income countries, such as Bangladesh, Haiti, India, Nepal, and Niger.

Room with a view
2 YEARS? ➕

If you're lucky enough to live or work in a pleasing environment—surrounded by gentle gardens, for instance—you'll know how much this counts toward providing a deep sense of well-being every day. Unsurprisingly, research has shown that after an operation, those patients who were assigned to hospital rooms with a pleasant outdoor view (of trees, for example) recovered faster and were discharged sooner than those who had a view of a brick wall.

Now, if a good view helps patients recover, it must surely help the rest of us keep healthy by lifting our mood, easing stress, and providing a deep sense of optimism and contentment. So park your chair by the window and take a good look outside. If you don't like what you see, put up posters or paint pictures on the wall—or just make sure you get out and spend some time every day somewhere where the view is good.

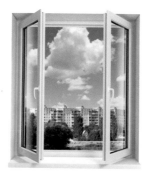

War zone

— 6 MONTHS

War can, and all too frequently does, take the lives of those who fight. But putting aside military deaths, civilians, too, suffer greatly reduced life expectancy. Every year spent living in a war zone could reduce your life span by about six months.

There are plenty of examples of the direct toll of war. It is estimated that nearly 10 million civilians died in World War I, while in World War II civilian deaths (35 million) outnumbered military deaths (25 million). The atomic bomb dropped in Hiroshima killed 80,000 innocent people in one blow; Agent Orange, the chemical weapon used during the Vietnam War, has for decades continued to wreak havoc on people's lives.

The indirect effects of war are even more significant, perhaps, regardless of where the conflict takes place: war uproots communities and destroys essential infrastructures such as hospitals, schools, and food and water supplies. Civilians forced to flee their homes lose their income and security, and are driven to live in squalid temporary shelters, where they suffer poor nutrition and a greater risk of disease.

The simple answer, of course, is that war is best avoided if you want a long and healthy life—unless you are an oppressed population for whom war brings liberation and improved conditions. In that case, perhaps, the right sort of war may extend life expectancy...

Heavily industrialized zones

2 YEARS —

It's a frightening prospect to think that the air you breathe could be killing you, but research has shown that living in the more industrial areas can affect life expectancy because of pollution in the air. The risk from pollution has been slowly improving thanks to UN Convention rulings which have, for example, cut sulfur pollution across Europe by two thirds in the past 25 years. But fine particles have escaped international control measures.

Polluting particles are released into the atmosphere when wood and fossil fuels are burned—clouds of them are emitted from the exhaust pipes of vehicles, for example. They can also form in the air from mixtures of pollutant gases. Larger particles fall quickly to the ground but fine particles stay in the air for much longer and can be carried by the wind long distances from their emission sources.

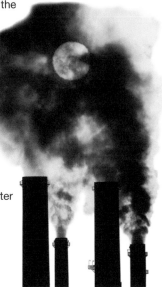

The World Health Organization has warned that a large number of health problems result from exposure to fine particles, which pass into the lungs when inhaled. Respiratory disease and cardiovascular disease can develop or be aggravated by the particle pollution.

So pack your bags for the countryside—or, better yet, start lobbying your government representative!

Free-radical damage

– **4 YEARS**

Our bodies are under a constant barrage of attack at a sub-microscopic level by free radicals—unstable atoms, essentially, that react with nearby compounds in order to regain stability—which exist both in our bodies and in the environment around us.

Within the body, free radicals are constantly being produced as part of various metabolic processes. Some of these have a purpose: the cells of the immune system generate free radicals, for example, in order to neutralize invading viruses and bacteria. But free radicals can also cause damage to the cell's own components, such as the DNA or genetic material, or the proteins in the cell membranes. The resulting cellular damage is a central mechanism in the aging process, as well as in diseases such as cancer, arthritis, cardiovascular disease, and Alzheimer's disease.

Environmental hazards—including radiation, and the chemicals in cigarette smoke, asbestos, coal, and herbicides—also increase our exposure to free radicals. Such environmental factors may provide an external source of free radicals or increase free-radical production by the body itself. It has been calculated that the DNA in each cell suffers about 10,000 free-radical "hits" every day. The lungs are particularly vulnerable to free-radical attack because many chemical pollutants are inhaled. But free radicals may also enter the body in the food we eat, or directly through the skin (as with radiation). Once in the body, the free radicals may trigger a sequence of activation of enzymes, inflammation, and release of chemical signals, which harms the tissues.

People who age well may have less oxidative free-radical damage. On the Japanese island of Okinawa, where people seem to be particularly long-lived, research shows that people following traditional ways of life have lower blood levels of free radicals, possibly because of healthier lifestyles but also because of genetic variations that give them greater protection. To counteract the effect of free radicals, the body uses antioxidants—molecules that safely react with the free radicals to limit damage. But as we get older our antioxidant processes become less efficient, resulting in our need to actively take in extra antioxidant nutrients (see entry 33).

How to limit free-radical damage

- Reduce environmental exposure.

- Avoid traffic exhaust fumes, which are high in cadmium.

- Steer clear of cigarette smoke (both first- and second-hand smoke).

- Reduce exposure to synthetic chemicals such as insecticides.

- Avoid heavy metals such as mercury, cadmium, and lead. Look out specifically for lead from old paint and pipes, high mercury levels in some fish (such as swordfish, tilefish, shark, and king mackerel), sewage sludge, fertilizers, pigments, and battery fluid.

- Avoid ionizing radiation from industrial pollution, sun exposure (see entry 63), cosmic rays, and medical X-rays.

- Reduce production of free radicals in the body by avoiding high-fat, high-sugar, over-processed foods.

- Increase intake of antioxidant nutrients.

Sunshine

✚ 2 YEARS

We know enough these days about skin damage to slather on the sunblock and retreat from the sun, but in doing so, many people are now missing out on a vital ingredient for long life—vitamin D.

The body uses sunlight to make vitamin D; it uses, more specifically, the ultraviolet B (UVB) ray—the type of UV that causes burning and that is the major target for sunblock.

Meanwhile, vitamin D helps protect against a host of life-shortening conditions, including many common cancers, multiple sclerosis, rheumatoid arthritis, hypertension, cardiovascular heart disease, and Type 1 diabetes. Without sufficient vitamin D, the muscles become weak and the risk of falls and fractures spirals, especially in older people. For some people, lack of sunlight, especially in the winter, can lead to mood changes and depression, known as Seasonal Affective Disorder (SAD).

What is needed is a balance: enough UVB to enjoy its health benefits but not so much that it damages the skin. You will need to take into account season, latitude, time of day, and your skin pigmentation in order to work out what is right for you. But a rough guide to sensible exposure is 10 to 15 minutes of sun on the arms and legs, or the hands, arms, and face, two times a week, ideally avoiding the hours of maximum intensity of sunshine (that is, between 12 p.m. and 2 p.m.).

Sunbathing

1 YEAR? —

The main risk from sunbathing comes from the increase in skin cancers when people are exposed to intense UV light. The pigmented skin cancers called melanomas are the most sinister: they are aggressive, spread easily, and can be difficult to treat.

The photoaging effect of UV light—and UVA rays—are significant if you want to retain a youthful look. A suntan is really a sign of the burning of the epidermis (top layer of skin). With continued exposure to the sun, skin becomes thinner and more fragile, and its connective tissues weaken, reducing strength and elasticity. Skin damage shows up in deep wrinkes, fine veins across the cheeks and nose, and patches of pigmentation such as tiny freckles and "liver spots." These are hard to avoid but you can limit or slow the damage by protecting your skin from excessive doses of UV light.

How to protect your skin from the sun

- Slip on suitable clothing.

- Slap on a wide-brimmed hat or stay in the shade.

- Slop on high-protection sunblock liberally, and reapply frequently.

- Avoid the strongest sun in the middle of the day.

- Avoid such intense UV that you get sun-burn, especially in childhood.

- Avoid sunbeds and lamps.

- Get all strange spots and moles checked out early (see entry 84).

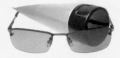

Radiation awareness

+ **1 YEAR**

The earth is naturally radioactive, as is the air you breathe, the food you eat, and the ground you stand on. Modern technology adds to the radiation bank new risks from sources such as X-ray machines, nuclear power stations, and even everyday objects such as smoke detectors and photocopiers.

There are two kinds of radiation we need to know about that can shorten a lifespan: ionizing radiation—which causes chemical changes that can damage living tissue—and non-ionizing radiation, which includes low-energy electromagnetic radiation (from power lines and cell phones, for example) and microwave radiation (see entry 66).

Ionizing radiation is used in radiotherapy treatment to kill cancer cells—so sometimes controlled radiation can help people to live longer. But usually it does harm, altering the way cells grow, function, or reproduce. Very large doses of radiation can cause tissues with a rapid cell turnover to die, resulting, for example, in skin burns, anemia, and loss of gut membranes. This may be rapidly fatal. More relevant are the long-term effects from chronic exposure, the most important of which is an increased risk of cancer, especially lung and blood cancer (leukemia).

Natural sources account for 85 percent of ionizing radiation. These include the earth's crust, from which seeps radon (see entry 65), which is responsible for half of all radiation exposure. Also, rocks, soil, and building materials, from which emanate gamma rays. Food and drink are another source of radiation because plants and animals take in radioactive materials with nutrients. Some foods such as brazil nuts, tea, coffee, and bread are more radioactive than others. Humans are also a potential source of radiation through our consumption of radioactive food and drink.

The sun and outer space, from which radiate cosmic rays, are normally shielded from us by the atmosphere, but at higher altitudes, where the air is thinner—in the mountains, for instance—we are susceptible to a bigger dose of these rays. Similarly, when you fly in a plane, you receive up to 100 times as much radiation as at sea level.

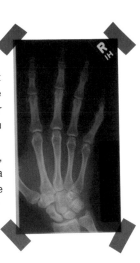

There are also important artificial sources of radiation, including medical tests and treatments, such as X-rays. On a larger scale, power stations, which release radioactive materials into the environment in gases (nuclear power) or ash (coal-fired power) are a source, as are nuclear power stations which discharge radioactive waste. But in reality the risk of your exposure to radiation from power and nuclear stations is very small, even if you live right next to them.

How to protect yourself from ionizing radiation

- Avoid unnecessary exposure.

- Reduce exposure to radon (see entry 65).

- Don't have unnecessary X-rays.

- Limit the number of flights you take or trips to high altitudes.

- Be aware of any exposure through your job and take appropriate steps to fix this. Research has shown, for example, that pilots who have clocked more than 5,000 flying hours may be at increased risk of acute myeloid leukemia due to cosmic radiation at high altitudes.

- Know the risk from your local environment—be aware, for example, of any local industries releasing radioactivity into the rivers or air.

Radon exposure
— **1 YEAR**

About 50 percent of the radiation that we are exposed to comes from radon, a natural radioactive gas that seeps out of the earth's crust and into our homes and offices. Radon is made by the radioactive decay of uranium, which is found throughout much of the earth's crust, but particularly in higher levels and in certain geological strata, especially in granite.

Levels indoors are usually low, but in areas rich in granite and uranium, larger amounts of the gas may permeate into buildings through cracks in the floor, or through the walls, if local granite building materials have been used. People in such areas may receive 5 or more times as much radiation from radon as the average. Long-term exposure to high levels of radon has been linked to an increased risk of lung cancer, especially among smokers.

How to reduce your risk from radon

- Check local radon levels. In high-level areas, get your home measured. Ask your local government representative about this—it may be a free service.

- If necessary, make simple changes to the ventilation system. An extractor fan beneath the building can reduce radon levels; in new buildings, an extensive damp-proof membrane across the full footprint of the building may be a cheaper option.

- If you are a smoker in a high-radon area you increase your risk dramatically, so stop smoking immediately.

Electromagnetic radiation
6 MONTHS? ▬

Electromagnetic radiation consists of electromagnetic waves produced by the movement of electrically charged particles. Examples include radio waves, microwaves, visible light, and X-rays. This type of non-ionizing radiation is given out by all modern electronic devices.

To what extent electromagnetic radiation is harmful to health, and a threat to longevity, is highly controversial. There is enough research to suggest that there is a risk, but how much of a risk, to whom, and in what situations isn't exactly clear. Many people are concerned about the risk from devices such as cell phones and their towers, microwave cookers and electricity lines. However, experts cannot agree whether living under power cables might increase leukemia or cell phone use increase the risk of brain cancer. Though epidemiological evidence suggests a higher rate of disease such as cancer in those people exposed to non-ionizing radiation, no study so far has been able to establish that this actually is the cause of the disease, or prove a mechanism for how the link might work. It's possible that electromagnetic fields act to concentrate other cancer-causing agents such as radon.

Until stronger evidence becomes available, your best bet may be to steer clear of non-ionizing radiation as far as is practical.

Reduce chemical use

+ **2 YEARS**

We come into contact with thousands of different chemicals every day, in the food we eat and the cleaning products we use, in pesticides, packaging, toys, medicines, and clothes, to name but a few items.

Although most cleaning products are labeled with known risks, other products in widespread use continue to cause problems ranging from allergies and asthma to infertility and a disruption of hormone levels. Seemingly innocuous activities may involve potentially hazardous chemicals: fill up with gas, for example, and the fuel vapors at the pump will give you a dose of hundreds of potentially toxic hydrocarbons and additives, including benzene, which is known to be linked to leukemia. Or renovate your 1960s home and you may risk breathing in asbestos fibers from the building materials, which could cause a form of lung cancer.

In the quest for a healthy lifestyle and a prolonged life span, you'll want to be aware of the chemicals in your environment and the risks they pose, as well as what you can do to reduce your exposure. Ecologically friendly or organic products may be the best way through our modern, chemically tinged world.

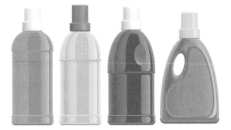

Noise pollution

1 YEAR

Turn down the sound or tug on some ear muffs—noise pollution is a significant factor contributing to the premature death of people throughout the world. According to research from the World Health Organization (WHO) Working Group on the Noise Environmental Burden of Disease, thousands of people lose years of healthy life as a result of the insidious effects of chronic noise exposure.

One of the most important links is between noise and the developed world's number-one killer, heart disease. Long-term exposure to traffic noise has been blamed for as many as 3 percent of deaths from coronary heart disease, or more than 200,000 deaths each year around the world. Noise creates a type of chronic stress which puts the body into a state of raised alert. Even when you are asleep, your brain and body continue to react to sounds, pumping out stress hormones, such as cortisol and epinephrine. These hormones can cause changes to the heart and blood vessels which contribute to high blood pressure, heart failure, heart attacks, and stroke. The threshold for cardiovascular problems is a chronic noise exposure of 50 decibels or above (just a little less than you would expect in a busy restaurant.)

Meanwhile, low-level background noise all around the clock, which most people recognize as irritating and depressing, can raise stress levels and may be responsible for just as many early deaths. A mere 35 decibels of background noise is enough to annoy and raise the risks. And nighttime noise may have an impact through its disruptive effects on sleep, so increasing fatigue, irritability, and aggression.

Dangerous parasites
— 2 YEARS

Hugging an animal may be good for your blood pressure (see entry 17), but it could also prove hazardous to your health. Next time you're feeding your racing pigeons, playing with your neighbor's friendly newts, or out strolling in the deer park, think of the hordes of microscopic wildlife that live, out of sight, on animals. Although the "host" animals themselves often seem quite healthy, they may be harboring dangerous microorganisms, including bacteria, viruses, fungi, and parasites. These organisms are able to jump ship to humans, either through direct contact or via food and water, and cause all sorts of trouble.

Deer ticks, for example, may migrate to the human body, carrying with them a bacterium that could cause Lyme disease. This can affect many systems of the body, including the joints, nerves, and heart. Although rarely fatal, it can cause long-term disability if left untreated. Similarly, a bacterium among birds exists that can easily pass to humans, causing pneumonia that can result in a severe illness.

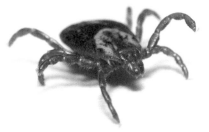

With salmonella from reptiles, worms and flukes from dogs, rabies from foxes, and flu from chickens and wild birds, there are plenty of good reasons to think twice before you get too close to an animal. Remember, too, to wash your hands after every encounter (see entry 72)!

Home safety

2 YEARS

Many of us worry about dying behind the wheel of a car and make an effort to drive safely, but chances are, you're actually more likely to die from an accident at home.

Fires, carbon monoxide poisoning, burns, falls, drowning, accidental collisions, and DIY accidents account for most at-home deaths. If you're about to undertake work on your house, be aware of the dangers involved, and make sure you complete the work to a safe standard. Even a simple thing such as falling off a step ladder may require hospital treatment.

When did you last safety check your home? Have you ever safety checked your home? Follow the list below to add years to your life.

How to be your own safety monitor

- Be aware of fire hazards, and remove them (see entry 74 for more).

- Check that your smoke alarm is in working order—don't forget to change the battery regularly.

- Know where the fire extinguisher is, and make sure it works.

- Make sure carpets are well secured and don't slip.

- Check that the wiring is sound.

- Ensure that doors are fitted with safety glass.

- If you have an elderly person in the house, install hand rails to help them move around safely.

Comfortable climate

+ 3 YEARS

The climate around us greatly influences many aspects of health and disease. At its extremes, cold weather brings the threat of exposure, hypothermia, and infections such as influenza, bronchitis, and pneumonia, while excessively hot weather can put intolerable strain on the heart, and cause problems with dehydration. The very old and very young are most vulnerable, especially when seasonal tolls such as influenza epidemics strike.

Somewhere in all this is the ideal climate, where the winters are mild and the summers are pleasantly warm. Sardinia may just represent the perfect spot. A remarkably high proportion of people who live there reach their century, including, unusually, a large number of men—there are 13.56 centenarians per 100,000 people in this balmy region. Or try Okinawa in Japan, where the temperature

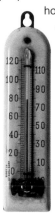

hovers around and above 68°F (20°C) for most of the year and, astonishingly, more than 40 out of 100,000 people are over 100 years old. The critical aspect in these places seems to be that many of those who reach the age of 80 proceed to survive for much longer—this is the stage at which we are most sensitive to the effects of climate and least able to cope with harsh conditions. Pack your bags now!

Washing your hands
2 YEARS

Only half of us wash our hands after visiting a public bathroom and, astonishingly, fewer than one in 10 doctors wash their hands between patients. Contact between people is the main way diseases spread. Even in diseases such as colds and flu, where we cough and sneeze viruses into the air, it is touching other people or their things, or holding door handles that are contaminated by others, that is the main route of transmission. Wash your hands, and you wash away the risk of disease.

How to wash your hands	When to wash your hands
• Wash with soap and clean running water for at least 20 seconds—and don't skimp on the soap! (Alternatively, use an alcohol-based cleaner and rub until hands are dry.) • Make a lather and scrub all surfaces of your hands, fingers and wrists. • Rinse hands well under running water. • Dry your hands on a paper towel, then use it to turn off the tap. Or dry with an air dryer.	• After using the toilet • Before and after changing a baby's diaper or potty-training a child • Before preparing or eating food • After blowing your nose or sneezing • Before and after looking after someone who is ill • Before and after treating a wound • After handing animals or their waste • After handling trash • After gardening

Workplace hazards

— 4 YEARS

Don't get down on your job just because it's boring. There are other things to worry about at the workplace—hazardous agents such as asbestos, dust, or industrial chemicals, for instance, or accidents and injuries from physically demanding work. Having a job linked to a known major industrial disease could reduce your life expectancy by four years.

Different jobs bring different hazards—and varying effects on one's life span. A radiographer working in the hospital X-ray department is exposed to different risks (such as radiation) than a metal industry worker (who, through exposure to metal dust, has a higher rate of lung cancer) or a miner (who, after years of inhaling coal dust may suffer from the progressive lung disease, pneumoconiosis). Disease may appear years after exposure or from second-hand exposure—some women have developed fatal asbestosis from shaking out and washing their construction-worker husband's work clothes, giving themselves a dose of microscopic asbestos dust.

Talk to your manager or your health and safety representative at work to be informed of the potential risks associated with your job, and what steps you or your employer should be taking to reduce those risks. Your personal health record, as well as other factors such as your genetic make-up, will influence how great these risks are. For example, certain people are genetically disposed to the development of asthma when working with industrial chemicals or metals. Arm yourself with the facts before you apply for a job, and then avoid those occupations with particularly deleterious health risks (see entry 98).

Fire protection

1 YEAR

Would you know what to do if a fire swept through your home, if your campfire raged out of control, or if your car burst into flames? Knowing what to do could mean the difference between life and death. Even if you can escape the flames, it's the smoke that kills most people, especially in house fires.

Walk through your house and think about how and where a fire might start. Ask a friendly firefighter to accompany you if you know one, or ask your local fire station if they'll send one over. And try to make your home as safe from fire as possible. Fire could kill you before your time. Don't let it.

How to fire-proof your home

- Don't let the batteries in your smoke alarms go dead.

- Check that all electrical appliances have been recently serviced, and that no wires are coming loose.

- Check that you aren't overloading any one system—for example, by plugging the TV, stereo, computer, and video game station into the same socket.

- Don't leave candles burning unattended.

- Switch off electrical items when you go to bed.

- Ensure you have a fire blanket close to hand in the kitchen, in case a fire starts at the stove.

Very few people would merely want to exist for a very long time, irrespective of what sort of condition they were in, or what they were able to do. The idea of becoming a pickled brain in a jar, with a few wires connecting our minds to the rest of the world, belongs firmly in the realm of science fiction movies. Most of us want to live longer in order to enjoy the world around us and the things we've worked hard to achieve—family, homes, a degree of success or wealth. To do this we need to be in reasonably good health—able to get around and take part in activities or conversations, and simply do what we want to do without every action being a struggle against disease, pain, and infirmity.

The term "health expectancy" allows us to think more closely about what we want to achieve when we strive for a longer life. Health expectancy refers to the expected years of life spent in good or fairly good health. While life expectancy has been increasing steadily, health expectancy is not increasing so fast. In other words, most of us can expect our health to decline as we get older.

If you want to live longer, you probably also want to stay healthy. This section looks at the steps you can take not just to extend your life but also to keep at bay (or under control) particular diseases such as high blood pressure, diabetes, or arthritis, which threaten to destroy the quality of your life even if they may not cut it short.

PART FOUR

Coping with Disease

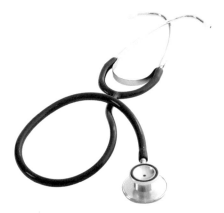

Vaccination

+ # 2 YEARS

Adults are often vulnerable to the same infectious threats children are—no matter what your age, vaccination will help you to live a longer life: you could gain two extra years if you routinely check with your doctor about the need for adult vaccines. The side effects of vaccinations are generally minimal and major problems very rare—they are certainly rarer than the risk from the disease you are being vaccinated against.

If you haven't already had the standard childhood vaccines such as measles, mumps, diphtheria, whooping cough (pertussis), or polio, talk to your doctor to see which ones you might need. Adults may be just as vulnerable to the effects of many of these infections; in fact, some of them cause a much more severe illness if caught in adult life.

Routine child immunizations

An immunization program from two months to 13 years would include:

- Diptheria

- Tetanus

- Whooping cough (pertussis)

- Measles and Mumps

- Polio

- Influenza and Chicken Pox

- Haemophilus influenzae tybe b (Hib)

- Rubella

- Meningitis

- Hepatitis A and B

- Pneumococcal

Adults need a tetanus vaccination, for example, just as much as children do, and should have a booster dose every 10 years. This disease (also known as lockjaw) is found all over the world and may be fatal in up to 20 percent of cases. Gardeners should be particularly careful to keep their tetanus immunization up to date—tough, resistant spores of the bacteria that cause tetanus (Clostridia) are found in the soil, and enter the body through any wound or scratch that punctures the skin.

People who travel frequently also need to make sure they are fully vaccinated against the infections that pose a risk in the country they are visiting. For example, vaccination against typhoid is not routine in the USA, but visitors to South Africa, where the disease is common, may well be advised to get vaccinated.

Vaccination against influenza becomes particularly important as we grow older. Because the flu virus constantly mutates, it's impossible to build up complete immunity to the disease. So everyone is vulnerable whatever their age or however many times they have had flu. In fact, older people may be more vulnerable because they have concurrent problems such as heart or lung disease.

In addition, everyone over age 65 and adults with chronic disease need a pneumonia vaccine, which protects against a common form of pneumonia-causing bacteria. These people need a revaccination every 10 years. New vaccines may dramatically affect life expectancy in the future. A vaccine that offers protection against human papilloma viruses (HPV, the cause of cancer of the cervix and other genital cancers) is now available, and many other anti-cancer vaccines are in the pipeline.

Take your pills

✚ 12 YEARS

Medicines can have a dramatic effect on keeping disease at bay and prolonging both health and life expectancy. Your doctor will prescribe a drug based on a sound knowledge of what benefits it can bring. But many medicines, especially those for chronic problems such as diabetes or high blood pressure, usually need to be taken carefully, as prescribed, every day for the rest of your life. People often forget or can't be bothered about their pills, or can't cope with the side effects but don't go back to their doctor to talk about the problem. As many as 25 percent of prescriptions for medicines are never taken to the pharmacy to be filled, and even when they are, many more are just left on the shelf at home and never taken as recommended.

A study of heart attack survivors in Toronto, Canada, showed a higher death rate for those patients who were particularly bad at taking their medicines after the attack.

But you don't need a scientific study to tell you that your prescribed pills aren't doing you any good just sitting in their bottles!

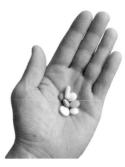

Side effects

4 YEARS ▬

Every single chemical you put in your body in order to achieve a desired effect (and this includes not just prescription medicines but herbal treatments, and recreational drugs such as cigarettes and alcohol) can have undesired effects or adverse, unexpected reactions. A drug that lowers your blood pressure nicely may cause insomnia, dizziness, or bring on headaches. Aspirin may keep the blood flowing smoothly, hence reducing the risk of stroke and heart attack, but it can also cause fatal stomach bleeds.

A study from the Netherlands has shown that nearly one in 50 admissions to hospital are for serious reactions to medication, and 6 percent of these are fatal. In the USA in 2000, there were an estimated 7,000 deaths among hospital patients due to medication errors, and 106,000 deaths simply due to the negative effects of medication. Research has also shown that the more medicines you need to take, the greater the chance that there will be a medical error of some sort. Older people taking three or four drugs a day are more than twice as likely to make a mistake; if you need seven medicines each day, the risk of errors is tripled.

Always read labels of your medicines and follow the instructions meticulously. Never double dose or take medicines prescribed for someone else. And get back to your doctor immediately if things don't seem right.

Regular screening

+ 4 YEARS

The principle is simple: the earlier you catch a disease, the less damage it is likely to have done, and the easier it should be to treat. As a result it should have less impact on health expectancy or longevity. Yet we often dismiss symptoms, delay getting expert advice, or hope the problem will go away. It's important to be vigilant for curious symptoms such as odd lumps and bumps, strange pains, rashes, the appearance of blood where it shouldn't be, or other changes in your body. Get advice from your doctor sooner rather than later about anything that is worrying you.

That said, many conditions march along deep inside the body without giving any clues to their existence—a small tumor in the intestines, perhaps, or blood rushing through your vessels under extraordinarily high pressure. Undetected, a tumor may spread to the liver where it is more resistant to treatment, or the high pressure of blood may rip through the vessels to cause a devastating stroke. The only way to pick up the first stages of a number of conditions is to regularly screen ostensibly healthy people for early signs of them.

For example, among every 100 of the many smokers blithely strolling around unaware that they have very high blood pressure, 10 will suffer a heart attack and five a stroke within the next five years. If they spent 60 seconds every year or two with a blood pressure machine wrapped around their arm (for that's about all screening for high blood pressure involves), their risk would be spotted, treatment could be started and many of the deaths or much of the possible disability avoided.

These are some of the screening tests you may want to talk to your doctor about. It is worth pointing out that screening can cause a lot of unnecessary worry about disease, especially when the tests used are not very sensitive, or produce false positive results which must be followed up with more invasive, potentially harmful tests that often show that there was nothing to worry about in the first place. So listen closely to the recommendations of your doctor—he or she can advise you on details such as how effective the test is, when it should be done, and how often it should be repeated.

Important screening tests

- Cancer

- Breast cancer: genetic testing, mammogram, physical examination

- Prostate cancer: prostate specific antigen (PSA) blood test, rectal examination

- Cervical cancer: pap smear, DNA testing for high-risk types of human papilloma virus

- Colon cancer: fecal occult blood (FOB) test, colonoscopy

- Ovarian cancer: genetic testing, pelvic examination, ultrasound scan, CA-125 antigen blood test

- Blood pressure: regular blood pressure measurements

- Heart disease: EKG, exercise stress test, cholesterol test

- Diabetes: fasting blood sugar levels

- Thyroid disease: thyroid hormone levels in blood

- Kidney disease: kidney function blood test and urine analysis

- Stomach and duodenal ulcers: helicobacter infection test in breath, blood or feces

- Glaucoma and other visual problems: dilated eye exam and pressure test

Risk of infection

— **1 YEAR**

The bubonic plague of the fourteenth century is one of the best-known epidemics and it killed an estimated one in four in Europe; smallpox is another. What the two have in common is the way they spread—rapidly, and through densely populated areas. Measles, influenza, polio, cholera, and dozens of other "crowd" diseases have more recently caused havoc among groups of people living together in close communities. As children we are often taught how "coughs and sneezes spread diseases," and we are encouraged to keep our germs to ourselves and keep a distance from others who are ill. But it's hard to avoid the infectious diseases that rapidly circulate when people gather together in semi-closed circumstances. Norwalk virus-induced gastroenteritis may swirl through the passengers on a cruise ship, meningococcal meningitis might break out among new students settling in a university dormitory, or a flu epidemic could make its mark on a retirement home. When there are a lot of humans around there is bound to be trouble.

If you live or work in close quarters with a lot of other people, you need to be particularly alert for the risk of infection, quick to keep away when illness starts spreading, and ready to visit your doctor immediately for advice and preventative medicines or early treatment.

Healthy partners

2 YEARS? +

The state of your health as you get older is influenced to a considerable degree by the health of your partner, as well as the rest of the family, so you'll want to make sure you and your partner keep an eye on each other's health.

Illnesses can be transmitted between partners during close contact or simply while sharing the same environment. Many infections, such as colds and mild gastroenteritis, are minor and short-lived. But others, such as meningitis, hepatitis, or HIV, can have a profound effect on health and life expectancy.

An illness in the family also places a social and economic burden on those family members who are not sick. A chronic illness can lead to a loss of income that may have major implications for the family: a fall in income, status, living conditions, and life satisfaction that the whole family will experience are all linked to shorter life expectancy.

Among elderly couples, the health of the "unit" (that is, both partners living together) may be essential in enabling them to support each other to live independently in their own home. It is often the case that when one of them becomes ill, the other struggles to cope without the mental and physical support of their partner, eventually becoming vulnerable to accidents and illness themselves.

Looking after your partner's health is all part of your own health agenda. Encourage your partner to follow the steps in this book, and make sure they seek help when things aren't right.

Heart disease

— **7 YEARS**

Disease of the heart and blood vessels (which together are known as cardiovascular disease) is the Number 1 killer in developed nations. Although statistics vary from country to country, cardiovascular disease causes serious problems for half the population of the Western world, and is to blame for about one in three deaths. According to the American Heart Association, life expectancy would increase by at least seven years if all forms of cardiovascular disease were eliminated.

Coronary artery disease (where the blood vessels to the heart are clogged) causes chest pain, shortness of breath, and heart failure, and can result in a heart attack. Stroke (damage to the brain as a result of disease of the blood vessels to the brain) may lead to terrible disability. Damage to the blood vessels elsewhere in

The polypill

In 2003, researchers at London's Wolfson Institute of Preventative Medicine proposed a "polypill" that contained six different drugs to lower the four key risk factors in cardiovascular disease. They said that the polypill should be given to everyone over the age of 55, and claimed that it could slash the rate of deaths from heart attack or stroke by more than 80 percent.

Those people who started taking it at 55, they said, could expect to gain an extra 12 years of life. The idea is based on more than 750 trials into the drugs, although the polypill itself is yet to be tested. Similar combination-drug treatments as an approach to prevention continue to be heavily debated.

the body can make exercise difficult and limit mobility. There is no doubt that cardiovascular disease shatters lives.

But there are many things that you can do to prevent cardiovascular disease, or reduce your risk of a heart attack or stroke even if you have already developed disease.

Start by stopping smoking (see entry 93), keep your blood pressure under control (see entry 88) and look at ways of reducing high cholesterol levels (see entry 36). It is also important to keep your size and shape healthy. An apple shape with a big tummy is particularly linked to cardiovascular disease. Measure your waist circumference rather than weight, and aim to keep it below 35 inches for women and 40 inches for men. You can help keep a healthy shape by exercising frequently. To protect your heart, you need only do 30 minutes of a moderate-intensity activity on most days of the week. But make sure you eat a healthy diet (see entries 28–38), otherwise all that exercise will go to waste. Another measure you can take is to ask your doctor about specific dietary supplements to boost the levels of essential micronutrients in your body—research has shown, for example, that the risk of heart disease is more than 30 percent lower among people with a high intake of folate or vitamin B_6. Not surprisingly, stress can also have a bad effect on your heart, so learn to deal with it (see entry 11). If you suffer from diabetes (see entry 87) it is important to manage this. And finally, ask your doctor about preventative medicines such as the polypill (see opposite page).

Bowel awareness

+ # 2 YEARS

If you want to live forever then you're going to have to abandon any inhibitions you might have about the business of your bowels. Making the top three on the list of common cancers, colon cancer still proves fatal in about 50 percent of cases, despite modern treatments. Not keeping an eye on what's going on down there could shave two years off your life.

Think first about the bowel-friendly changes that you may need to make to your lifestyle. Aim for a diet with less red and processed meat and a lot more vegetables and fiber, as well as a higher fish and milk intake. Regular physical activity and weight control are also important for keeping the bowel healthy.

Be alert to signs of trouble, especially if you have a family history of colon cancer. Ask your doctor about any applicable screening tests, like a colonoscopy, or scans of the abdomen. Meanwhile, research shows that sending off a fecal sample for testing every two years can reduce your risk of dying from colon cancer by 15 percent—a good return for a small, if rather unpleasant, task: about 50 percent of cancers detected this way are in the earliest stage, with a survival rate of greater than 80 percent.

And if you develop symptoms such as a change in a regular bowel habit, or passing blood or mucus in the toilet, then get advice from your doctor urgently.

Skin cancer awareness

1 YEAR +

Playing disease detective is quite straightforward when it comes to the skin. You'll need to look out for the pigmented skin cancers called malignant melanomas as these can be very aggressive, spread quickly, and have a high mortality unless caught very early. Malignant melanoma has been increasing faster than any other type of tumor since the suntan became fashionable. To decrease your risk of developing skin cancer, protect yourself from the harmful effects of UV light (see entry 63) and keep an eye on your skin.

How to examine your skin

It's important to check your own skin once a month. Self-examination is best done in a well-lit room in front of a full-length mirror.

- Check your face, ears, neck, chest, and belly. Women will need to lift breasts to check the skin underneath.

- Check both sides of your arms, the tops and palms of your hands, and your fingernails.

- Sitting down, first check one leg, then the other. Inspect the bottoms of feet, calves, and the backs of thighs.

- Use a hand-held mirror to inspect your neck, shoulders, upper arms, back, buttocks, and legs.

- Check for the following: A mole is more likely to be abnormal if a) one half of the mole does not match the other half; b) the edge of the mole is jagged or irregular; c) more than one color is present in the mole; d) it is larger than 5 mm in diameter.

Remember, thin melanomas are curable, so get to know your skin and moles well.

Cancer

— **3 YEARS**

Perhaps the main reason that a diagnosis of cancer is so feared is that it almost inevitably brings a threat of death. But the impact of cancer on life or health expectancy is hugely variable—you could lose a year or more of life expectancy for any sort of cancer other than non-pigmented skin cancer—and depends on factors such as the type of cancer, the location of the tumor, the age and general fitness of the patient, the treatment given, the expertise of the health professionals providing treatment, the occurrence of complications, and other co-incidental events.

Cancer of the pancreas, for example, is very aggressive and difficult to treat—only about 10 to 15 percent survive longer than a year after diagnosis, and only 2 to 3 percent are alive after five years. In comparison, survival rates in non-pigmented skin cancers are very high, and as many as 90 percent of people are cured and go on to enjoy a normal life expectancy.

Overall it is estimated that about one in three people will be diagnosed with some form of cancer at some stage in their life. But cancer is predominantly a disease of aging—below the age of 50 only about one in 27 people develop cancer. It becomes more likely as genetic damage accumulates over time, destroying the normal controls on cell division and growth. And as humans gradually live longer, so the proportion of people who develop cancer will increase.

How to reduce the risks of cancer

- Avoid the known triggers.

- Give up smoking cigarettes or a pipe, or chewing tobacco (entry 93).

- Avoid pollution and free radicals (entries 60 and 61).

- Avoid excess sun exposure (entry 63).

- Get more fruit and vegetables in your diet (entry 35).

- Get enough nutrients in the form of vitamins (entry 30), minerals (entry 37), and antioxidants (entry 33).

- Get plenty of fiber in your diet (entry 31).

- Exercise regularly (entry 41).

- Keep clear of radiation (entries 64–66).

- Take preventative medicines. Aspirin has been shown to significantly reduce the rate of new polyps in people both with and without a history of colon polyps. However, taking aspirin to lower cancer risk should not been regarded as a substitute for established prevention tactics such as fecal occult blood testing and colonoscopy.

- For women, get vaccinated against human papilloma virus. This sexually transmitted infection is strongly linked to cancer of the cervix, vulva, anus, and other sites.

- Try to catch cancer early.

- Check your body regularly (entries 82–86).

- Get expert advice on concerning symptoms.

- Go for screening (entry 78).

- Get the best treatment. Information is power if you are diagnosed with cancer: find out about different treatments and talk to your doctor.

Breast awareness

+ 1 YEAR

While breast screening with mammograms and other scans saves thousands of lives every year, a cancer may sometimes appear in between scans or before a woman first goes for a scan. Staying alert for early signs of a tumor could mean the difference between survival and death, because the earlier a tumor is spotted the less chance it has to spread and the easier it will be to treat. Do some of your own detective work: be attentive to how your breasts normally look and feel, for example by examining them once a week or so in the bath or shower (or while lying down quietly if this is easier), and learning how to spot any worrying changes. There is no such thing as a perfectly normal breast. Each woman's breasts look and feel different, especially at different times of the menstrual cycle, and at different ages and stages of life. In the days just before a period, for example, the breast can feel lumpy and sore, especially higher toward the underarms. Learn what is normal for you.

The majority of breast lumps are harmless but there is only one way to be sure — talk to your doctor about any changes you have noticed or are worried about. Signs to look out for include: changes in the shape of the breast or the position of the nipple (or the direction it points in — if a nipple inverts this should be checked out at once); dimpling, puckering or unusual thickening of the skin; different sensations in the breast or skin over it, including pain, heaviness, or numbness; and changes to the nipple such as itching, discharge, bleeding, crusting or a rash.

Although men are at much lower risk from breast cancer, they do have small amounts of breast tissue and can cancer can occur there or in the nipples, so they too need to be alert for the symptoms or signs.

Testicle check

6 MONTHS +

Screening programs aren't routinely used for testicular cancer, but you can take action yourself to reduce your risk simply by finding out about the symptoms and learning how to check for it. First, you've got to recognize your risk factors with the chances being greater for those who: have a relative who has had testicular cancer; have previous problems with an undescended testicle; tend to live a sedentary lifestyle; have had sexually transmitted infections or trauma to the testicle in the past; have a mother who smoked while she was pregnant; are Caucasian from northern European countries, such as Scandinavia and the UK.

Men aged 15 to 40 should perform a monthly self-examination, and get to know how their testicles usually look and feel. Self-examination can be very helpful in detecting the cancer in its early stages, when it has the best chance to be fully cured.

Important symptoms to watch out for:

- Any enlargement of a testicle
- A significant loss of size in one of the testicles
- A feeling of heaviness in the scrotum
- A dull ache in the lower abdomen or in the groin
- A sudden collection of fluid in the scrotum
- Pain or discomfort in a testicle or in the scrotum
- Enlargement or tenderness of the breasts

Diagnosis

—

5 YEARS

The degree to which diabetes can shorten life depends on a variety of factors, including the type of diabetes (whether it is Type 1 insulin-dependent diabetes, which tends to be more severe, or Type 2, which tends to be associated with adult onset and obesity), the age at which it is diagnosed, and whether you have other risk factors that add complications, such as heart disease. Poorly controlled diabetes could take five years off your average life expectancy.

In diabetes the body is unable to move sugar from the blood into the cells because of inadequate insulin supplies. Blood sugar levels rise while the cells must use alternative sources of energy. This wreaks damage on the blood vessels, including the coronary arteries supplying the heart. As many as 75 percent of people with diabetes develop cardiovascular disease as well. Diabetes also damages the nerves and can cause kidney failure and blindness. It leads to an increased susceptibility to infection and impaired immune function as well, leaving you less able to fight other diseases.

Diabetes: Know the risks

- Besides age and weight, what factors increase your risk for Type 2 diabetes?

- you have a parent, brother, or sister with diabetes.

- your family background is Alaska Native, American Indian, African American, Hispanic/Latino, Asian American, or Pacific Islander.

- you have had gestational diabetes, or have given birth to at least one baby weighing more than 9 pounds.

- your blood pressure is 140/90 mm Hg or higher, or you have been told that you have high blood pressure.

- your cholesterol levels are not normal. Your HDL cholesterol ("good" cholesterol) is below 35 mg/dL, or your triglyceride level is above 250 mg/dL.

- you are fairly inactive, exercising fewer than three times a week.

- you have polycystic ovary syndrome, also called PCOS (women only).

- you've had impaired glucose tolerance (IGT) or impaired false glucose (IFG).

- you have other clinical conditions associated with insulin resistance, such as acanthosis nigricans.

- you have a history of cardiovascular disease.

• Recognize symptoms. These include increased thirst, passing urine more frequently, weight loss, tiredness, blurred vision, hunger, and increased infections.

• Get diagnosed early. As many as one in three are unaware they have the condition, while high blood-sugar levels silently damage their tissues.

• Control your weight. If you are at high risk of developing diabetes, a 7 percent weight loss and 150 minutes of moderate-intensity exercise each week will halve that risk. Once diabetes is established, losing weight may help you to live longer. Researchers at the University of Surrey found that obesity in diabetics can reduce life expectancy by eight years.

• Take steps to reduce complications. Look after your heart (see Fac. 81), kidneys, eyes, and feet.

• If you have diabetes, the single most important thing you can do to minimize the risk that diabetes poses to longevity is to very tightly control the levels of glucose in the blood.

High blood pressure
— **5 YEARS**

High blood pressure, or hypertension, makes the heart work harder, damaging the blood vessels and increasing the risk of developing heart disease (see entry 81), as well as kidney disease and stroke. Once developed, it usually is a problem for the rest of your life, but until complications set in, there are typically no symptoms and people are unaware they have a problem.

The first step is to get your blood pressure measured regularly—many people don't even know what theirs is. Blood pressure is recorded as two numbers: the systolic pressure (as the heart beats and forces blood through the blood vessels—this is the higher number) over the diastolic pressure (as the heart relaxes). For example, a measurement would be written as 120/80 mmHg (millimeters of mercury). The optimum blood pressure rate is less than 120/80; a blood pressure of 121–139/80–89 is sometimes known as "prehypertension" because the person is likely to develop the condition in the future. A consistent blood pressure reading of 140/90 or higher is considered high blood pressure that usually needs medical treatment.

A long list of drugs is used to treat hypertension. They all have side effects but most are minimal and easily tolerated so work with your doctor to find one that suits you best, and take it regularly. But there are other things that you can do, too, on a daily basis, to help keep those blood pressure levels down. For instance, reduce salt intake, lose excess weight, exercise regularly, manage stress and look after your heart (see entry 81).

Arthritis

1 YEAR   —

Arthritis means inflammation of the joints, bones, and supporting tissue. There are more than 100 types but most common by far is osteoarthritis. If you looked closely at people over 60 you would find almost every single one had some degree of osteoarthritis. Osteoarthritis doesn't directly affect life expectancy because it is not in itself fatal. However, it has a profound effect on health expectancy, causing chronic pain and reduced mobility, interfering with a person's ability to exercise, disturbing their sleep patterns, and seriously reducing quality of life. Other types of arthritis such as rheumatoid arthritis—where, in addition to joint problems, one may suffer severe inflammation of other tissues, including the heart—may more directly impinge on longevity. While you might lose a year of your life if you suffered from moderate osteoarthritis, you could lose four years if you had severe immobilizing osteoarthritis.

How to reduce the risks of osteoarthritis

- Reduce excess weight so that your joints don't have to bear large loads.

- Do regular gentle exercise to help build up the strength, stability, and range of motion of your joints. But you should avoid doing high-impact exercise such as aerobics, which can put excessive strain on the joints.

- If you have osteoarthritis, ask your doctor about drug treatments such as non steroidal anti-inflammatory drugs that help to minimize joint damage. In more severe disease, aim to maintain mobility using drug treatments or, if it becomes necessary, surgery (joint replacements, for example).

Osteoporosis

— **3 YEARS**

As you age, your bones become less dense, and their internal scaffolding breaks down. This process, known as osteoporosis, makes the bones fragile and susceptible to a fracture. It's a particular problem in women, where it results from the decline in levels of female hormones that occurs after menopause. It has been estimated that osteoporosis will affect 15 percent of women at the age of 50, 30 percent at 70, and 40 percent at 80. Combined with an increasing weakness of the muscles and the failing sense of balance that occurs with age, osteoporosis creates a recipe for disaster. Many cases of falls in the elderley result in a fractured or broken bone, often the hip or a vertebra. The consequent immobility leads to muscle wasting, loss of confidence, and an increased risk of infections such as pneumonia.

How to keep osteoporosis at bay

- Build up your bones by getting the recommended daily amounts of calcium (1,000–1,300 milligrams) and vitamin D (400–800 IU) from a young age.

- Take dietary supplements if necessary.

- Do weight-bearing exercise (such as walking, running, tennis, or dancing) several times a week.

- Avoid smoking and excessive alcohol.

- From about age 65 (age 60, if you are at an increased risk of osteoporosis), go for bone density tests and take medication recommended by your doctor.

Looking young
1 YEAR? +

In a society where the dominant forces of media and advertising celebrate youth to such an extent that older people may find themselves marginalized, it takes an unusual inner strength (or lack of concern) to enthusiastically sport gray hair and wrinkles without a care in the world—especially if you are a woman. There is perhaps not such a big leap from streaking your hair purple when you were 17 to dying your hair at a later age to cover the gray; similarly, it may not be such an effort to accept a Botox injection or an eyelid lift if you have already accepted being pierced for earrings.

Whatever the moral issues of cosmetic surgery, the vast majority of people who choose to go under the surgeon's knife find it a positive experience. Though it may not prolong life, modern techniques mean the risks of routine surgery are small, so it is unlikely to shorten life. And if nothing else, the improvement in mood and self-esteem that most people feel when they achieve their goal to wipe off a few years from their looks, could add a little to life expectancy—it certainly can improve quality of life (see entries 1, 2, and 4 for possible psychological benefits from cosmetic surgery).

If you want to strive hard to look younger, go for it! Just a few simple rules: be careful to find a reputable surgeon; do your homework about what to expect; don't expect miracles; anticipate the risks and keep generally fit and healthy before and after surgery.

Dementia

— 5 YEARS

In order to stay well and live longer, we need to be able to look after ourselves, respond to sudden threats to our health, and understand and implement the long-term changes and actions that are needed to prevent or effectively fight disease. This requires brainpower. Sadly, dementia, a widespread problem throughout the world that becomes more common with advancing age, often slowly robs a person of their ability to care for themselves. Those afflicted with dementia withdraw from the world, eventually losing interest in eating, drinking, or moving, and become vulnerable to complications such as infection or falls. The disease also steals the enjoyment of life from many sufferers.

Dementia affects one in 20 people over 65, one in five over 80, and nearly one in two over 95. It can be viewed as a terminal disease because it is progressive,

Some "superfoods" that may help keep your brain healthy

- Blueberries may protect the neurons in the brain from oxidative stress and help prevent the decline seen in conditions such as Alzheimer's disease.

- Packed with Omega-3 oils (see entry 38), salmon helps to improve memory, while reducing inflammation in the body and protecting us from various age-re-lated conditions such as arthritis and heart disease.

- Broccoli contains a whole range of protective nutrients, including vitamin C, betacarotene, indole-3-carbinol (I3C), and sulphurophane (which can protect against cancer), and also seems to protect the brain against decline.

usually incurable, and limits life span. There are many different types of dementia and the prognosis varies, but in general the research shows that people usually live for only five to nine years after symptoms first occur.

You can take measures to reduce your risk. For instance, the common risk factors for cardiovascular disease are also a threat to the tiny blood vessels that feed the tissues of the brain. High cholesterol, diabetes, hypertension, and smoking during midlife are each associated with a 20 to 40 percent increase in the risk of dementia later on. So tackle these risk factors (see entries 36, 87, 88, 93.)

It is also important to avoid pollution, including other people's cigarette smoke: scientists at the University of California have found that people with a high lifetime exposure to second-hand smoke are about 30 percent more likely to develop dementia.

Also of benefit is learning. The higher the education level you achieve when young, the lower the risk of dementia later. And keeping your brain active as you get older—by learning new skills, for example—helps to prevent mental decline.

A final point is to make sure you are eating healthy foods. There is some suggestion that a diet full of antioxidants (entry 33) and fatty fish at least once a week may help prevent dementia. A lot of research is being carried out into other dietary elements—curcumin, the main active ingredient of turmeric, may possibly help against Alzheimer's, for example, while ginkgo biloba might improve memory and overall function in people with dementia.

Your first difficult decision, as a child, may have been choosing between orange or raspberry ice cream. But soon enough you find you're having to make decisions that can have a marked long-term effect on life and health expectancy, such as whether to try a cigarette or whether to have unprotected sex. The basis of a healthy lifestyle is to make the right choices so that you remain fit and well.

We all make dubious decisions or behave in a careless way now and then, but some people tend to intentionally choose more risky behavior than others do. Thriving on the adrenaline rush of living on the edge, these are the people who would rather snowboard down a mountain than take up golf, or experiment with drugs without a thought to the dangers.

Though people may be drawn to try something risky for a variety of reasons—peer pressure, for example, or simple curiosity—it turns out our genes may also be spurring us on. Unraveling the genetics behind risk-taking behavior, scientists have discovered that certain genetic make-ups may encourage more of a buzz in some people. Still, there is no genetic condition that completely removes free will. Even the most dedicated thrill-seeker is able to make a choice about which activity to undertake. It *is* possible to balance a healthier life with having fun.

PART FIVE

Choices and Risks

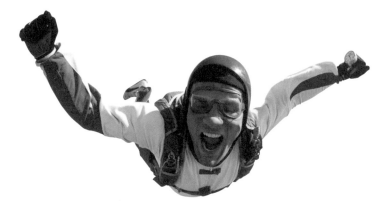

Smoking

— 8 YEARS

Cigarette smoking is the single most important cause of preventable disease and premature death in developed countries. Tobacco smoke contains over 4,000 chemicals, many of which are highly toxic, such as arsenic, formaldehyde, cyanide, benzene, toluene, and acrolein.

Because smoking increases the risk of at least 50 different medical problems—from cancer and heart disease to infertility, digestive problems, and dementia—it has a huge impact on health expectancy. Almost one third of all cancer deaths (including 90 percent of deaths from lung cancer), 80 percent of deaths from bronchitis and emphysema, and around 17 percent of deaths from heart disease (which together account for a large proportion of all deaths) are directly due to smoking. Lifelong smokers have only about a 50 percent chance of living past the age of 65, but even if they do reach old age it is likely to be blighted by chronic respiratory problems, cardiovascular disease, and a poor quality of life. About half of all smokers are killed by their addiction.

A study of British doctors in 2004, by R. Doll, R. Pet, J. Boreham, and I Sutherland, has found that those who smoked lost, on average, about 8 years of life. But those smokers who quit before middle-age had the same sort of life expectancy as non-smokers.

Smoking interferes with some of the basic pleasures of life. It can destroy appetite and enjoyment of food because it seriously affects taste and smell, and it increases the risk of impotence because it damages the blood supply to the sex organs. Smoking also accelerates the aging process—wrinkles and gray hair appear up to a decade earlier than might be expected if it weren't for a 20-a-day habit.

You can turn back the clock, though. Once smokers quit, their health risks rapidly drop, and within a few years they may almost be back to normal. For example, the risk of a heart attack for a quitter drops to the same level as a non-smoker's within three years. And giving up cigarettes usually leads to considerable savings, hence reducing financial worries and allowing ex-smokers to enjoy more healthy pleasures, such as vacations.

How to quit smoking and stay a non-smoker

- Believe you will be successful.

- Quit when you are in the right frame of mind. If you know you're having a bad week or are generally having trouble coping, it's not the right time.

- Don't go it alone—have a friend do it with you or join a smoking cessation program. With maximum support and effective medical treatments, up to 30 percent of people will not be smoking at the end of a year.

- Follow a structured plan—a smoking cessation clinic or program will help you create this.

- Make sure you have the necessary psychological support.

- Use medical treatments such nicotine-replacement therapy or anti-craving drugs as directed by your health professionals. These are proven to double your chances of success compared to psychological support alone. And if one form of nicotine replacement doesn't seem to help, try a different one.

- If your attempt to quit fails, don't give up. See the attempt as a milestone: learn from it what factors did or didn't work for you so that next time you will be successful.

Recreational drugs
— 4 YEARS

There is a real risk of danger even with so-called "recreational drugs" such as cannabis, which some argue is not very harmful. While cannabis doesn't directly cause deaths, scientists are slowly discovering the damage it can do. Cannabis smoke contains higher levels of cancer-causing substances than tobacco, and is inhaled for longer periods of time, for example. Research has shown that the highest risk of pre-cancerous abnormalities in the lung occurs when cannabis and tobacco are smoked together. Significant and long-lasting psychotic effects can also occur. But, perhaps most importantly, the drug often introduces a person to the culture of substance abuse, which leads down a slippery slope to more harmful drugs and greater risks.

The dangers of drugs such as cocaine and heroin are more widely appreciated, as well as the links with other harmful behavior such as crime (in order to pay for a drug habit) or transmission of infections such as HIV and hepatitis C through contaminated needles. The average life expectancy of heroin or morphine addicts is only about six to eight years. Even with treatment, their lives are shortened, on average, by about 15 years. Steer clear of recreational drugs if you want to maximize your health or life expectancy—the consequences can be devastating.

Red wine

3 YEARS +

Some years ago researchers noticed that the French, despite eating lots of fatty foods, have low rates of cardiovascular disease. Although they drank five times as much red wine as their neighbors in the UK, they were four times less likely to die from heart disease. Since then, several studies have shown that drinking one to two units of alcohol a day is linked with better health and a longer life. Data from various studies consistently show a reduction of about 20 percent in the risk of heart disease in people who drink about one unit of alcohol a day.

Research suggests that the polyphenolic compounds found in red wine interfere with the formation of atherosclerosis (fatty deposits that "harden" the arteries), helping to keep the blood vessels healthy. Many of these polyphenolic compounds have an antioxidant effect (see entry 33), which may explain why a moderate intake of alcohol could also be linked with a lower risk of cancer. Though the findings are still under discussion, a little tipple, ultimately, is unlikely to do you any harm, and could well help you live longer.

Know your units

One unit of alcohol is 0.3 ounces (8 grams) of alcohol and is typically described as:

- One small glass of wine; or

- Half a pint of any average-strength beer; or

- A bar or pub measure of spirits, such as gin or whisky

But drink strengths vary, as do pub measures and wine-glass sizes, so these are just a rough guide.

Binge drinking

—

3 YEARS

The discovery that the national habit of drinking red wine seemed to protect the French from heart disease overlooked a key fact—far more men in France (and elsewhere) die from the harmful consequences of drinking alcohol than might be saved by its beneficial effects. While a little might do us good, there's no doubt that alcohol in any great measure is a poison that can harm most of the systems of the body: exceeding recommended alcohol limits more than once every two weeks could well reduce your life expectancy by three years.

And doctors are now learning how binge drinking—drinking large amounts of alcohol in a matter of hours or over a long weekend—may be particularly harmful even when a person's overall alcohol intake is within recommended limits.

After just a few drinks, alcohol starts to take its toll on the brain, causing degeneration of the delicate brain cells. The sensory cells for smell may be among the most sensitive to an alcohol binge but damage to other areas of the brain swiftly follows. There are detectable impairments in memory, and reactions are slowed, making accidents more likely. A sense of relaxation progresses into a loss of inhibitions, and blackouts may occur as more is drunk. After an alcohol soaked night out on the town, tissues throughout the body pay the price. The brains of adolescents—the people most likely to binge drink—seem to be particularly vulnerable to alcohol damage. Women are also more sensitive to the effects.

Perhaps the most notorious effect of chronic alcohol intake is on the liver, where it causes inflammation of the liver cells, called hepatitis, and scarring, a condition called cirrhosis. But it also causes stomach ulcers, and inflammation of the stomach and the pancreas. Alcohol interferes with absorption of nutrients in the intestines, and can lead to osteoporosis or thinning of the bones. It damages the muscle of the heart, and the nerves and brain, leading to memory problems,

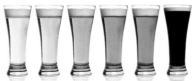

depression, and dementia. Impotence is common in heavy drinkers, and a large alcohol intake may contribute to infertility. Alcohol also increases the risk of cancer of the mouth, esophagus, liver, colon, and breast.

And if it doesn't get your body it may yet affect the rest of your life: alcohol is a frequent factor in problems with family, relationships, work, finances, and crime. It's easy to see how drinking heavily can take years off your life.

How to drink more safely

- Stick to recommended limits: most experts advise no more than three to four units of alcohol a day for men and no more than two to three units a day for women.

- Don't drink during pregnancy.

- Don't give alcohol to children.

- Don't consume your entire week's allowance of units in one evening. Binge drinking, which produces very high levels of alcohol in the body, is far more toxic to the cells than if the same amount of alcohol were to be consumed at a slower, steadier rate, say over the course of a week.

- Never drink and drive.

- Try not to drink on an empty stomach. Food can help slow absorption of alcohol into the blood.

- If you are worried about how much you drink or suspect you may be dependent on or addicted to alcohol (if you need alcohol first thing in the morning to face the day, for example) get expert advice or talk to your doctor.

Adventure travel

2 YEARS

Travel abroad can be deeply enriching but the price for adventure may be a significant risk to life and limb. There are hundreds of potential dangers out there, from unpleasant tropical diseases that could make you very ill to unfamiliar customs and conventions that might land you in trouble with the law. Developed nations such as the USA and those in Europe and Australasia usually seem fairly safe, but accidents and illness can happen anywhere—especially if you travel unprepared for danger. In destinations all over the world, vacationers' troubles range from robberies to traffic accidents, from sunstroke to food poisoning. And when you're thousands of miles from home and struggling with a medical, legal, or social support system that is different from what you're used to, it may be difficult to know who to turn to for help.

How to travel safely

- Do your homework before you go—learn about and prepare for the risks.

- Find out about vaccinations and medical needs.

- Take out full travel insurance.

- Make sure people at home know where you are going and how to contact you.

- Act responsibly and respect the culture and customs of the countries you visit.

Crazy careers
3 YEARS

When you think about dangerous jobs what comes to mind may be stuntmen, bomb disposal experts, and high-wire walkers. But a study by researchers at Oxford University found that some of the most dangerous jobs are on the ocean waves, where adverse weather conditions, accidents, and collisions are major hazards. The study found fishermen and -women at greatest risk, with merchant sailors coming a close second. It was found that people working on the sea are up to 50 times more likely to die while working, compared to those in other jobs. On average, of every 100,000 fishermen, 103 will die at work—this is up to 50 times higher than the average job. Crab fishing in the icy Bering sea was especially hazardous. Only timber cutters fare worse, with 118 per 100,000 dying, mostly when their trees fall onto them.

Take a look at life or car insurance statistics, too, and you'll find actors, rock stars, and comedians paying some of the highest premiums. While the jobs themselves may not be inherently dangerous, the lifestyle involved is often so erratic and pressured, and the rates of alcohol and drug abuse so notoriously high, that the risks to health and life expectancy outnumber those of almost any other career.

If you really want to be cautious, apply to be an insurance clerk, a domestic cleaner, a supermarket cashier, or a call center worker—the Oxford study confirmed that these sorts of service-sector jobs are the safest, with death rates of just 0.7 per 100,000 workers.

Extreme sports

— 5 YEARS

Being active is an essential ingredient in any recipe for living longer. But if your choice of exercise is racing head-first down the Cresta Run on a skeleton toboggan then it could also be your downfall. While the thrill of an adventurous sport may offer that feel-good factor, a serious accident could also dramatically shorten your life. Injury is an ever-present risk in most sports. The Consumer Product Safety Commission in the US estimates that the highest numbers of sport-related injuries are from basketball (over 400,000 serious injuries a year), football (the average age at death for an NFL pro is 55 years), and bicycling. In Australia, motorsports, horse riding, and power boating are the most dangerous, according to researchers at Monash University in Australia. And insurance companies levy the heaviest penalties on those who fly planes, climb mountains, hang glide, parachute, scuba dive, or take part in motorsports.

How to get active—safely

- Go slowly and don't jump in at a level beyond your experience or capabilities. Work your way up to more adventurous activities.

- Always get expert advice and training.

- Wear the proper clothing, and use the proper equipment and safety gear.

- Follow the rules.

- Don't play if you are injured.

Road safety

3 YEARS +

In 1896, at Crystal Palace in London, UK, 44-year-old Bridget Driscoll became the first person in the world to be knocked down and killed by a car. Today, more than a million people are killed on the roads every year, and up to 50 million are injured. Road traffic accidents are now the leading cause of violent deaths and injuries worldwide—and many of the victims are young. They are more likely than any disease to cause death or disability to those between the ages of 5 and 40.

Details about the driver of the car that knocked down Mrs. Driscoll provide some clues about why road traffic accidents happen even now. He had been driving for only three weeks, and even these days, drivers new to the roads still have a much higher accident rate. Edsell was said to have altered the car to make it go faster than it should; today, "boy racers" driving poorly modified souped-up cars at high speed are still a major risk. Edsell was also distracted by talking to the young woman in the passenger seat beside him; distractions—whether from passengers, music, cell phones, or something lost in the driver's mind—still play a part in many accidents.

No matter how safely you drive you may still be at the mercy of some other careless driver. But if you drive within the speed limit, in a well-maintained car, unaffected by alcohol, and concentrating solely on the road and traffic, you have a better chance of getting out of a tricky situation alive.

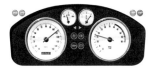

Conclusion

I hope this book has inspired you and left you feeling optimistic that it is possible to take your fitness and well-being into your own hands. You should now have a better understanding of where the threats lie to achieving a long life, as well as how much time you may be able to buy if you manage to control or fend off these threats. The world around us is packed with a myriad of thrilling experiences—stimulating sights and sounds, awe-inspiring views, breathtaking activities—that you can enjoy into old age; it would be a terrible waste to check out early while you are still enjoying yourself.

But you should also have gained a sense of the work involved in trying to live forever. Many of the easy options in life are the least healthy choices, and you may have to start asking yourself some uncomfortable questions about the decisions you've made about your lifestyle. To achieve a long life, it's usually necessary to look beyond the quick rewards and invest in a way of life that slowly brings longer-term benefits.

Along the way you're going to need some good help, support, and information, so listen closely to the comments and advice of those around you. Think about what your friends, family, or colleagues say but don't take any of it as the gospel truth, even if they are a top heart surgeon. There are very few simple black and white facts in health, and most medical advice must be weighed up in the context of any individual's own life and medical background.

Beware hype—there's a lot of misinformation out there, much of it disguised as publicity for some new miracle eating plan or wacky therapy that's completely unproven and likely to empty your wallet faster than it can turn back your body's clock. Double-check specific medical information by playing detective in the library (an underrated wealth of health information) or on the Internet. Use your common sense and instincts to sift opinion from fact, then work out what might be right for you. Finally, talk to a friendly doctor, nurse, or other health professional to get the full low-down.

Some particularly good sources for sound and practical health advice are the Internet sites run by national health institutions or governmental bodies (full websites below). The National Institutes of Health has very thorough information (health.nih.gov), especially at Medline Plus. You might also find it useful to look at the websites of renowned institutions such as the Mayo Clinic (www.mayoclinic.com). In addition, of course, there are hundreds of other good websites (including www.deathclock.com and www.realage.com), books, patient support groups, and expert resources—including your own doctor.

So start taking action to stop that slide into decrepitude. You, too, could live forever... almost!

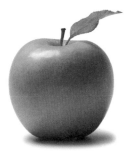

Resources

PART ONE

2. Happiness

Audrain J., Schwartz M., Herrera J., et al. "Physical activity in first degree relatives of breast cancer patients." *Journal of Behavioral Medicine* 2001; 24:587–603.

Cohen S., Doyle W.J., Turner R.B., et al. "Emotional style and susceptibility to the common cold." *Psychosomatic Medicine* 2003; 65:652–657.

Diener E., Seligman M.E.P. "Beyond money: toward an economy of well-being." *Psychological Science in the Public Interest* 2004; 5(1):1–31.

http://www.psych.uiuc.edu/~ediener/hottopic/1-31.pdf.

Lox C.L., Burns S.P., Treasure D.C., Wasley D.A. "Physical and psychological predictors of exercise dosage in healthy adults." *Medicine and Science in Sports and Exercise* 1999; 31:1060–1064.

Vitaliano P.P., Scanlan J.M., Ochs H.D., et al. "Psychosocial stress moderates the relationship of cancer history with natural killer cell activity." *Annals of Behavioral Medicine* 1998; 20:199–208.

3. Optimism

Fitzgerald T.E., Prochaska J.O., Pransky G.S. "Health risk reduction and functional restoration following coronary revascularization: a prospective investigation using dynamic stage typology clustering." *International Journal of Rehabilitation and Health* 2000; 5:99–116.

Kamen-Siegel L., Rodin J., Seligman M.E., Dwyer J. "Explanatory style and cell-mediated immunity in elderly men and women." *Health Psychology* 1991; 10:229–235.

Kubzansky L.D., Sparrow D., Vokonas P., Kawachi I. "Is the glass half empty or half full? A prospective study of optimism and coronary heart disease in the normative aging study." *Psychosomatic Medicine* 2001; 63:910–916.

Maruta T., Colligan R.C., Malinchoc M., Offord K.P. "Optimism-pessimism assessed in the 1960s and self-reported health status 30 years later." *Mayo Clinic Proceedings* 2002; 77:748-753.

Maruta T., Colligan R.C., Malinchoc M., Offord K.P. "Optimists vs. pessimists: survival rate among medical patients over a 30-year period." *Mayo Clinic Proceedings* 2000; 75:140–143.

5. Conscientiousness

Schwartz J.E., Friedman H.S., Tucker J.S., et al. "Sociodemographic and psychosocial factors in childhood as predictors of adult mortality." *American Journal of Public Health* 1995; Sept 85(9):1237–45.

Terman L.M., et al. *Terman Life-cycle Study of Children with High Ability* 1922–1986. [Computer file]. 2nd release. Palo Alto, CA: Robert R. Sears [producer], 1986. Ann Arbor, MI: Inter-university Consortium for Political and Social Research 1989.

6. Having faith

Koenig H. (Ed.) *A Handbook of Religion and Mental Health* Burlington, Mass.: Academic Press (1998)

7. Marriage

Cameron P., Cameron K., Playfair W.L. "Does homosexual activity shorten life?" *Psychological Reports* 1998;83(3 Pt1):847–66.

Gardner J., Oswald A. "How is mortality affected by money, marriage and stress?" *Journal of Health Economics* 2004; 23(6):1181–1207

http://www2.warwick.ac.uk/fac/soc/economics/staff/faculty/osw ald/mortalitymarchos2004.pdf.

Kaplan R.M., Kronick R.G. "Marital status and longevity in the United States population." *Journal of Epidemiology and Community Health* 2006; 60(9):760–5.

8. Divorce

Ambert A.M. *Ex-spouses and New Spouses: a study of relationships* Greenwich, CT: JAI Press 1989.

Bloom B.L., Asher S.J., White S. "Marital disruption as a stressor: a review and an analysis." *Psychological Bulletin* 1978; 85:867–94.

Coombs R.H "Marital status and personal well-being: a literature review." *Family Relations* 1991.

Engstrom G., Khan F.A., Zia E., Jerntorp I., Pessah-Rasmussen H., Norrving B., Janzon L. "Marital dissolution is followed by an increased incidence of stroke." *Cerebrovascular Disease* 2004; 18 (4):318–24.

Goodwin J.S., Hunt W.C., Key C.R., Sarmet J.M. "The effect of marital status on stage, treatment, and survival of cancer patients." *Journal of the American Medical Association* 1987; 258:3125–30.

Hetherington M.E., Kelly J. *For Better or For Worse: Divorce Reconsidered*. New York, NY: W.W. Norton & Company 2002.

Kposawa A. "Divorce and suicide risk." *Journal of Epidemiology and Community Health* 2003; 57:993.

Marks, N.F., Lambert J.D. "Marital status continuity and change among young and midlife adults: longitudinal effects on psychological well-being." *Journal of Family* 1988; 19:652–86.

Price S.J., McKenry P.C. *Divorce* Beverly Hills, CA: Sage.1988.

Weiss R.S. "The impact of marital separation." In: Levinger G.,

Moles O.C., (Eds.), *Divorce and Separation: Context, causes, and consequences*. New York, NY: Basic Books. 1979.

9. Young mothers

Hawkes K. "Human longevity: The grandmother effect." *Nature* 2004; 428:128–9.

Helle S., Lummaa V., Jokela J. "Are reproductive and somatic senescence coupled in humans? Late, but not early, reproduction correlated with longevity in historical Sami women." *Proceedings. Biological Sciences/The Royal Society* Jan 7 2005; 272(1558): 29–37.

Smith K.R., Mineau G.P., Bean L.L. "Fertility and post-reproductive longevity." *Social Biology* Fall–Winter 2002; 49(3–4)185–205.

10. Community

http://www.biomedcentral.com/1471-2458/5/65.

11. Stress

Herbert, J. "Stress, the brain, and mental illness." *British Medical Journal* 1997; 315:530–5.

Holmes, T.H., Rahe, R.H. "The social readjustment rating scale." *Journal of Psychosomatic Research*, 1967; 11:213–218.

Horowitz, M., Schaefer, C., Hiroto, D., Wilner, N., Levin, B. "Life event questionnaires for measuring presumptive stress." *Psychosomatic Medicine* 1977; 39(6):413–431.

14. Exercise

http://www.hno.harvard.edu/gazette/1998/06.04/AlumsFindSecret.html.

Audrain J., Schwartz M., Herrera J., et al. "Physical activity in first degree relatives of breast cancer patients." *Journal of Behavioral Medicine* 2001; 24:587–603.

Lee I.M., Paffenbarger Jr. R.S. "Associations of light, moderate, and vigorous intensive physical activity with longevity. The Harvard Alumni Health Study." *American Journal of Epidemiology* Feb 2000; 151(3):293–9.

Lox C.L., Burns S.P., Treasure D.C., Wasley D.A. "Physical and psychological predictors of exercise dosage in healthy adults." *Medicine and Science in Sports and Exercise* 1999; 31:1060–4.

16. Laughter

Martin R.A. "Humor, laughter, and physical health: methodological issues and research findings." *Psychological Bulletin* Jul 2001; 127(4):504–19.

17. Pets

Allen K., Blascovich J., Mendes W.B. "Cardiovascular reactivity and the presence of pets, friends, and spouses: the truth about cats and dogs." *Psychosomatic Medicine* Sept–Oct 2002; 64(5):727–39.

Friedmann E., Thomas S. A. "Pet ownership, social support, and one-year survival after acute myocardial infarction in the Cardiac Arrhythmia Suppression Trial (CAST)." *American Journal of Cardiology* Dec 1995; 15:76(17):1213–7.

Siegel J.M. "Stressful life events and use of physician services among the elderly: the moderating role of pet ownership." *Journal of Personality and Social Psychology* 1990; 58(6):1081–6.

18. Depression

Clarke S.P., Frasure-Smith N., Lesperance F., Bourassa M.G. "Psychosocial factors as predictors of functional status at 1 year in patients with left ventricular dysfunction." *Research in Nursing and Health* 2000; 23:290–300.

Faller H., Kirschner S., König A. "Psychological distress predicts functional outcomes at three and twelve months after total knee arthroplasty." *General Hospital Psychiatry* 2003; 25:372–373.

Miller G.E., Cohen S., Herbert T.B. "Pathways linking major depression and immunity in ambulatory female patients." *Psychosomatic Medicine* 1999; 61:850–60.

Spiegel D., Giese-Davis J. "Depression and cancer: mechanisms and disease progression." *Biological Psychiatry* 2003; 54:269–82.

Zorrilla E.P. et al. "The relationship of depression and stressors to immunological assays: a meta-analytic review." *Brain, Behavior, and Immunity* 2001; 15:199–226.

Zorrilla E.P., Redei E., DeRubeis R.J. "Reduced cytokine levels and T-cell function in healthy males: relation to individual differences in subclinical anxiety." *Brain Behavior, and Immunity* 1994; 4:293–312.

19. Meditation

Walton K.G., Schneider R.H., Nidich S.I., et al. "Psychosocial stress and cardiovascular disease part 2: effectiveness of the transcendental meditation program in treatment and prevention." *Behavioral Medicine* 2002; 28(3):106–23.

20. Active mind

Wilson R.S., Mendes De Leon C.F., Barnes L.L., et al. "Participation in cognitively stimulating activities and risk of incident Alzheimer disease." *Journal of the American Medical Association* Feb13 2002; 287(6):742–8.

Wilson R.S., Scherr P.A., Schneider J.A., Tang Y., Bennett D.A. "The relation of cognitive activity to risk of developing Alzheimer's disease." *Neurology* Jun 27 2007.

PART TWO

21. Long living parents

Gross L. "The key to longevity? Having long-lived parents is a good start." *Public Library of Science Biology* April 2006; 4(4):119.

Iwata K., et al. "Aging-related occurrence in Ashkenazi Jews of leukocyte heteroplasmic mtDNA mutation adjacent to replication origin frequently remodeled in Italian centenarians." *Mitochondrion* Jul 7 2007; (4):267-72.

22. Only child

Krzyzanowska M., Boryslawki K. "Number of siblings and children of short and long living individuals." *International Journal of Anthropology* 2002; 17(3–4):173–80.

Penn D.J., Smith K.R. "Differential fitness costs of reproduction between the sexes." *Proceedings of the National Academy of Sciences USA* 2007; 104(2):553–8.

23. Bad genes

http://elegans.uky.edu/300_Spr06/Aging_Spr06_Lect14.pdf.

Barbieri M., Bonafè M., Franceschi C., Paolisso G. "Insulin/IGF-I-signaling pathway: an evolutionarily conserved mechanism of longevity from yeast to humans." *American Journal of Physiology: Endocrinology and metabolism* 2003; 285(5):1064–71.

Cawthon K., Smith E., O'Brien A., et al. "Association between telomere length in blood and mortality in people aged 60 years or older." *The Lancet* 2003; 361(9355):393–5.

Lio D., Scola L., Crivello A., et al. "Gender-specific association between -1082 IL-10 promoter polymorphism and longevity." *Genes and Immunity* 2002; 3(1):30–3.

Niemi A.K., Moilanen J.S., Tanaka M.A., et al. "A combination of three common inherited mitochondrial DNA polymorphisms promotes longevity in Finnish and Japanese subjects." *European Journal of Human Genetics* 2005; 13(2):166–70.

Willcox B.J., Willcox D.C., He Q., et al. "Siblings of Okinawan centenarians share lifelong mortality advantages." *The Journals of Gerontology. Series A, Biological sciences and medical sciences* (J Gerontol A Biol Sci Med Sci) 2006; 61:345–54.

24. Girls rule!

http://www.news.harvard.edu/gazette/1998/10.01/WhyWomenLiveLon.html.

http://www.incore.ulst.ac.uk/about/specialist/cyms/CYMS_ru1.pdf.

http://www.statistics.gov.uk/cci/nugget.asp?id=1092.

http://www.statistics.gov.uk/articles/hsq/hsq 32-injury&poisoning.pdf.

25. Stay short

Samaras T.T. "Storms LH. Impact of height and weight on life span." *The Bulletin of the World Health Organisation* 1992; 70(2):259–67.

26. Obesity

Adams K.F. *New England Journal of Medicine* 2006;355:758–759, 763–778, 779–787.

27. Being underweight

http://news.bbc.co.uk/2/hi/health/4606011.stm.

28. Eating less

Mattson M.P. "Neuroprotective signaling and the aging brain: take away my food and let me run." *Brain Research* 2000; 886(1–2):47–53.

Mattson M.P., Duan W., Guo Z. "Meal size and frequency affect neuronal plasticity and vulnerability to disease: cellular and molecular mechanisms." *Journal of Neurochemistry* 2003; 84(3):417–31.

Morgan T.E., Wong A.M., Finch C.E. "Anti-inflammatory mechanisms of dietary restriction in slowing aging processes." *Interdisciplinary Topics in Gerontology* 2007; 35:83–97.

31. Fiber

American Heart Association Conference on Cardiovascular Disease Epidemiology and Prevention (Mar 2 2007) http://www.americanheart.org/presenter.jhtml?identifier=3045797.

Cade J.E., Burley V.J., Greenwood D.C. "Dietary fibre and risk of breast cancer in the UK Women's Cohort Study." *International Journal of Epidemiology* 2007; 36(2):431–8.

Kromhout D., Bloemberg D.P., Feskens E.J. "Alcohol, fish, fibre and antioxidant vitamins intake do not explain population differences in coronary heart disease mortality." *International Journal of Epidemiology* 1996; 25(4):753–9.

Obrador A. "Fibre and colorectal cancer: a controversial question." *British Journal of Nutrition* 2006; 96(Supplement No.1):S46–S48.

33. Antioxidants

Clarke R., Armitage J. "Antioxidant vitamins and risk of cardiovascular disease. Review of large-scale randomised trials." *Cardiovascular Drugs and Therapy* (sponsored by the *International Society of Cardiovascular Pharmacotherapy*) 2002; 16(5):411–5. http://www.ahrq.gov/clinic/3rduspstf/vitamins/vitcvdsum2.htm.

34. Fast food

http://www.newscientist.com/article.ns?id=dn9318&feedId=online-news_rss20.

35. Mediterranean diet

http://www.bbc.co.uk/health/health_over_50/gettingolder_facts.shtml.

37. Minerals

http://dietarysupplements.info.nih.gov/factsheets/magnesium.asp.

Akbaraly N.T., Arnaud J., Hininger-Favier I., et al. "Selenium and mortality in the elderly: results from the EVA study." *Clinical Chemistry* 2005; 51(11):2117–23.

Pawelec G., Ouyang Q., Wagner W., et al. "Pathways to a robust immune response in the elderly." *Immunology and Allergy Clinics of North America* 2003; 23(1):1–13.

38. Omega-3s

Simopoulos A.P. "Essential fatty acids in health and chronic

disease." *American Journal of Clinical Nutrition* 1999;
70(3):560S–569S.

39. Bad posture
Kado D.M., Huang M.H., Karlamangla A.S., et al.
"Hyperkyphotic posture predicts mortality in older
community–dwelling men and women: a prospective study."
Journal of the American Geriatrics Society 2004; 52(10):1662–7.

41. Getting active
http://www.hno.harvard.edu/gazette/2001/05.31/01-exercise.html.
Lahmann P. "Cancer epidemiology biomarkers and prevention."
Stroke 1998; 29:2049–54.
Franco O.H., et al. "Effects of physical activity on life expectancy
with cardiovascular disease." *Archives of Internal Medicine* 2005;
165(20):2355–60.
Lee I.M., Sesso H.D., Oguma Y., Paffenbarger R.S. Jr. "The
'weekend warrior' and risk of mortality." *American Journal of
Epidemiology* 2004; 160(7):636–41.

43. Balance
Gillespie L.D., Gillespie W.J., et al. "Interventions for preventing
falls in elderly people." *Cochrane Database of Systematic
Reviews* 2003; 4.

44. Couch potato
http://mednews.stanford.edu/stanmed/2002summer/shorttake_l
iving.html.
Myers J., Prakash M., Froelicher V., et al. "Exercise capacity and
mortality among men referred for exercise testing." *New
England Journal of Medicine* Mar 14 2002; 46:793–801.
Vaughan C. "Living on the couch is living on the edge." *Stanford
Medicine Magazine* 2002.
Wannamethee S.G., Shaper A.G., Walker M., Ebrahim S.
"Lifestyle and 15-year survival free of heart attack, stroke, and
diabetes in middle-aged British men (British Regional Heart
Study)." *Archives of Internal Medicines* 1998; 158(22):2433–40.

45. Not getting enough sleep
http://www.pnas.org/cgi/content/full/103/38/13901#F1#F1.
Cirelli C. "Sleep disruption, oxidative stress, and aging: new insights
from fruit flies." *Proceedings of the National Academy of Sciences
of the United States of America* 2006; 103(38):13901–02.
Tafaro L., Cicconetti P., et al. "Sleep quality of centenarians:
cognitive and survival implications." *Archives of Gerontology and
Geriatrics* 2007; 44S:385–9.

46. Napping during the day
http://science.nasa.gov/headlines/y2005/03jun_naps.htm.
Newman A.B., Spiekerman C.F., Enright P., Lefkowitz D.,
Manolio T., Reynolds F., Robbins J. "Daytime sleepiness
predicts mortality and cardiovascular disease in older adults."
Journal of the American Geriatrics Society 2000; 48(2):115–23.
Stiles S., "Untreated obstructive sleep apnea may worsen
survival in heart failure." *Heartwire* April 6 2007
http://www.medscape.com/viewarticle/554749.

48. Good dental hygiene
The American Academy of Periodontology 2005 "Tooth or
consequences: 10 steps to add years to your life."
http://www.perio.org/consumer/addyears.htm.
Beck J. et al. "Periodontal disease and cardiovascular disease."
Journal of Periodontology 1996; 67(suppl 10):1123–37.

49. Good sex
Abramov L.A. "Sexual life and frigidity among women
developing acute myocardial infarction." *Psychosomatic
Medicine* 1976; 38:418–25.
Butler S.M., Snowdon D.A. "Trends in mortality in older women:
findings from the nun study." *Journal of Gerontology* 1996; Ser
B 51:S201–8.
Kaplan S.D. "Retrospective cohort mortality study of Roman
Catholic priests." *Preventive Medicine* 1988; 17:335–43.
Leitzmann M.F., Platz E.A., Stampfer M.J., et al. "Ejaculation
frequency and subsequent risk of prostate cancer." *Journal of
the American Medical Association* 2004; 291:1578–86.
Palrnore E.B. "Predictors of the longevity difference: a 25-year
follow-up." *Gerontologist* 1982; 6:513–8.
Persson G. "Five-year mortality in a 70-year old urban
population in relation to psychiatric diagnosis, personality,
sexuality and early parental death." *Acta Psychiatrica
Scandinavica* 1981; 64:244–53.
Smith G.D., Frankel S., Yarnell J. "Sex and death: are they
related? Findings from the Caerphilly cohort study." *British
Medical Journal* 1997; 315(7123):1641–4.

54. Frequent pregnancies
Confidential Enquiry into Maternal and Child Health "Why
mothers die 2000–2002: Report on confidential enquiries into
maternal deaths in the United Kingdom."
http://www.cemach.org.uk/publications/WMD2000_2002/
content.htm.
Conde-Agudelo A., Belizán J.M. "Maternal morbidity and
mortality associated with interpregnancy interval: cross sectional
study." *British Medical Journal* 2000; 321:1255–59.

55. Hormone replacement
Mayoclinic.com "DHEA: Anti-aging supplement has no benefit,
study finds." http://www.mayoclinic.com/health/dhea/HA00083.
Writing Group for the Women's Health Initiative Investigators
"Risks and benefits of estrogen plus progestin in healthy
postmenopausal women: principal results from the Women's
Health Initiative Randomized Controlled Trial." *Journal of the
American Medical Association* 2002; 288(3): 321–33.

PART THREE

56. Place of birth

http://news.bbc.co.uk/1/hi/health/263033.stm.

57. City life

Gartner A., Gibbon F., Riley N., "A profile of rural health in Wales." *Wales Centre for Health*
http://www.wales.nhs.uk/sites3/page.cfm?orgld=568&pid=24302.

General Register Office for Scotland "Life expectancy in special areas (urban/rural, deprivation and community health partnerships) in Scotland, 2003–2005."
http://www.gro-scotland.gov.uk/statistics/publications-and-data/life-expectancy/life-expectancy-in-special-areas-2003-05/main-points.html.

Takano T., Nakamura K., Watanabe M. "Urban residential environments and senior citizens' longevity in megacity areas: the importance of walkable green spaces." *Journal of Epidemiology and Community Health* 2002; 56:913–8.

peopleandplanet.net "The Urban Millennium."
http://www.peopleandplanet.net/doc.php?id=2805.

58. Room with a view

Diener E., Seligman M.E.P. "Beyond money: toward an economy of well-being." *Psychological Science in the Public Interest* 2004; 5(1):1–31.
http://www.psych.uiuc.edu/~ediener/hottopic/1–31.pdf.

Lee I.M. Lee, et al. "Exercise intensity and longevity in men. The Harvard Alumni health study." *Journal of the American Medical Association* 1995; 273(15), Apr 19.

59. War zone

Centers for Disease Control and Prevention National Vital Statistics Reports 54(14)
http://www.cdc.gov/nchs/data/nvsr/nvsr54/nvsr54_14.pdf.

Globalis "El Salvador: life expectancy at birth."
http://globalis.gvu.unu.edu/indicator_detail.cfm?Country=SV&IndicatorID=18.

Sandova J. "Civil war and the effect on life expectancy: El Salvador." http://www.josesandoval.com/2007/04/civil-war-in-el-salvador-and-effect-it.html.

World Resources Institute "Population, health, and human well-being - El Salvador." *EarthTrends*
http://earthtrends.wri.org/pdf_library/country_profiles/pop_cou_222.pdf

60. Heavily industrialized zones

Convention on Long-range Transboundary Air Pollution of the United Nations Economic Commission for Europe (UNECE)
http://www.unece.org/env/lrtap/

United Nations Economic Commission for Europe "Keeping air pollution in check can add two years to your life."
http://www.unece.org/press/pr2004/04env_p18e.htm

61. Free radical damage

Ames B.N., Shigenaga M.K., Hagen T.M., et al. "Oxidants, antioxidants, and the degenerative diseases of aging." *Proc Natl Acad Sci USA* 1993; 90:7915–22.

62. Sunshine

Holick M.F. "Vitamin D: important for prevention of osteoporosis, cardiovascular heart disease, type 1 diabetes, autoimmune diseases, and some cancers." *Southern Medical Journal* 2005; 98(10):1024–27.

Holick M.F. "Sunlight and vitamin D for bone health and prevention of autoimmune diseases, cancers, and cardiovascular disease." *American Journal of Clinical Nutrition* 2004; 80 suppl. 6:1678S–88S.

64. Radiation awareness

Health Protection Agency "High Radon Houses found in Cornwall."
http://www.hpa.org.uk/hpa/news/nrpb_archive/press_releases/2004/press_release_08_04.htm

International Commission on Non-Ionizing Radiation Protection
http://www.icnirp.de/

Nuclear Industry Association "Radiation, health and nuclear safety."
http://www.niauk.org/radiation-and safety.html#What_is_radiation

UK Independent Expert Group on Mobile Phones
http://www.iegmp.org.uk/

67. Reduce chemical use

European Commission "Environment Fact Sheet: REACH—A new chemicals policy for the EU."
http://ec.europa.eu/environment/chemicals/reach/fact_sheet.pdf.

London Hazards Centre "Asbestos in the home—part 1."
http://www.lhc.org.uk/members/pubs/factsht/56fact.htm.

69. Dangerous parasites

Health Protection Agency "Table of Zoonotic Diseases."
http://www.hpa.org.uk/infections/topics_az/zoonoses/table.asp.

71. Comfortable climate

Okinawa Centenerian Study "Okinawa's Centenarians."
http://okicent.org/cent.html

72. Washing your hands

Handwashing Liaison Group. "Hand washing: a modest measure with big effects." *British Medical Journal* 1999; 318:686.

Tibballs J. "Teaching hospital medical staff to handwash." *Medical Journal of Australia* 1996; 164(7): 395–8.

Weeks A. "Why I don't wash my hands between each patient contact." *British Medical Journal* 1999; 319:518.

73. Home safety

BBC News Online "Home hazards 'kill more than cars'." Mar 20 2001. http://news.bbc.co.uk/1/hi/health/1230176.stm.

74. Fire protection

Watson L., Gamble J. "Fire Statistics, United Kingdom 1998" http://www.fire.org.uk/advice/FA/odpm_fire_601423.pdf.

76. Take your pills carefully

Starfield B. "Is US health really the best in the world?"*Journal of the American Medical Association* 2000; 284(4):483–5.
Van der Hooft C.S., et al. "Adverse drug reaction-related hospitalisations: a nationwide study in the Netherlands." *Drug Safety* 2006; 29(2):161–8.

81. Heart disease

Law M.R., Wald M.J., Morris J.K., Jordan R.E. "Value of low dose combination treatment with blood pressure lowering drugs: analysis of 354 randomised trials." *British Medical Journal* 2003; 326:1427 http://www.British.Medical. Journal.com/cgi/content/full/British Medical Journal; 326/7404/1427.
Law M.R., Wald M.J., Rudnicka A.R. "Quantifying effect of statins on low density lipoprotein cholesterol, ischaemic heart disease, and stroke: systematic review and meta-analysis." *British Medical Journal* 2003; 326:1423http://www.British Medical Journal.com/cgi/content/full/British Medical Journal;326/7404/1423.
Rodgers A. "A cure for cardiovascular disease?" *British Medical Journal* 2003; 326:1407–8.
Wald N.J., Law M.R. "A strategy to reduce cardiovascular disease by more than 80%." *British Medical Journal* 2003; 326:1419 http://www.BritishMedicalJournal.com/ cgi/content/full/British Medical Journal;326/7404/1419.

83. Skin cancer awareness

Lens M.B., Dawes M. "Global perspectives of contemporary epidemiological trends of cutaneous malignant melanoma." *British Journal of Dermatology* 2004; 150:179–85 http://www.medscape.com/viewarticle/470300.

84. Cancer

New England Journal of Medicine 2003; Mar 6;348(10): 879–80, 883–90, 891–9.

88. High blood pressure

InCirculation.net "Hypertension shortens life expectancy." http://www.incirculation.net/18471_51773.aspx?usechannel=.

87. Diabetes

BBC News Online "Obesity cuts diabetic life span." Mar 17 2004 http://news.bbc.co.uk/1/hi/health/3517294.stm.

Centers for Disease Control and Prevention "National Diabetes Fact Sheet." http://www.cdc.gov/diabetes/pubs/pdf/ndfs_2005.pdf

90. Osteoporosis

Bandolier "Outcome after hip fracture." http://www.jr2.ox.ac.uk/ bandolier/band49/b49-5.html.

92. Dementia

Canadian Study of Health and Aging http://www.csha.ca/ Whitmer R.A., Sidney S., Selby J., Claiborne-Johnston S., Yaffe K. "Midlife cardiovascular risk factors and risk of dementia in late life." *Neurology* 2005; 64:277–81. http://www.neurology.org/cgi/content/abstract/64/2/277

93. Smoking

Doll R., Richards P., Boreham J., Sutherland I. "Mortality in relation to smoking: 50 years' observations on male British doctors." *British Medical Journal* 2004; 328:1519.
Hughes J. R., Shiffman S., Callas P., Zhang J. "A meta-analysis of the efficacy of over-the-counter nicotine replacement." *Tobacco Control* 2003; 12:21–7.

94. Recreational drugs

Smyth B., Fan J., Hser Y.I. "Life expectancy and productivity loss among narcotics addicts thirty-three years after index treatment." *Journal of Addictive Diseases* 2006; 25(4):37–47.

96. Binge drinking

Gaffney J. "Light to moderate wine drinkers live longer, according to Dutch report." *Wine Spectator* Mar 2 2007 http://www.winespectator.com/Wine/Features/ 0,1197,3677,00.html.
Law M., Wald N. "Why heart disease mortality is low in France: the time lag explanation." *British Medical Journal* 1999; 318:1471–80 http://www.British Medical Journal.com/cgi/content/ full/318/7196/1471.

97. Adventure travel

"Risky business." http://blogs.guardian.co.uk/travelog/ 2006/07/risky_business.html

98. Crazy careers

"Dangerous jobs." http://www.menatrisk.org/health/ dangerousjobs.html

100. Road safely

"World's first road death" http://www.roadpeace.org/articles/worldfir.html

Index